The Care Gaps

W. Halamandaris

UNIVERSITY
PRESS OF
AMERICA

pdm

Lanham • New York • London

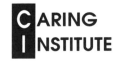

CARING INSTITUTE

Copyright © 1992 by
University Press of America®, Inc.
4720 Boston Way
Lanham, Maryland 20706

3 Henrietta Street
London WC2E 8LU England

Co-published by arrangement with the
Caring Institute

Library of Congress Cataloging-in-Publication Data

Halamandaris, W., 1945–
The care gaps / W. Halamandaris.
p.   cm.
1. Medical policy—United States.   I. Title.
RA395.A3H34   1992   362.1'0973—dc20   92–6438 CIP

ISBN 0–8191–8658–9 (cloth : alk. paper)
ISBN 0–8191–8659–7 (pbk. : alk. paper)

For my brother, Val, who has taught me most of what I know.

The Care Gaps

Contents

Preface

—— ❦ ——

If past is prologue, this book will create controversy.

There are about ten million Americans who are fed by the medical-industrial complex. Over the years, we have done something to offend most of them.

People have lost jobs, families, and fortunes as a result of our work. People have been indicted, convicted, and gone to jail. Some have died as a result of our investigations.

Companies have gone bankrupt. Executives, accustomed to the kind of respect that accompanies position and power, have found themselves being cross-examined by congressional panels and making guest appearances on "60 Minutes," "20/20," or the evening news.

Not surprisingly, as the years wore on, some of these good people began to take a considerable interest in our health and welfare. With some regularity, some lawyer, lobbyist, or other professional liar would try to make their mark by getting us fired. They tried going over our heads. They tried party politics, organized dissenting opinions, encouraged minority reports, and contributed like relatives.

A few found more creative means of expressing their displeasure. My brother has been sued at least eight times for a total approaching $400 million. He's won each contest, but each time he has wondered if he will have to hock the house to pay the lawyers, and his wife talks about putting the family silver in her name. His house has been burglarized and his life threatened.

For whatever reason, I am generally treated somewhat more kindly. People who don't know me and have no particular reason to like me have offered to set me up in business, find me soft company, and give me other things I didn't know I needed. One of them was kind enough to leave a gas can in my garage early one morning. Unfortunately, he departed before I could thank him.

A couple of years ago when we released a report that described in detail the various ways half a dozen large corporations were banging our government, the leader of the pack reciprocated by inviting me to down to Texas. He said something about going fishing in the Gulf. Since his company had lost close to $100 million on the market the day our report was released, I didn't bother to ask if I should bring my own gear.

One of the New York sharpies had a similar thought and took me on a joy ride through some of the more picturesque parts of the Bronx. While we surveyed the territory, he explained who his friends were and how they did business. Meanwhile his dog, a rather large German Shepherd, sat between my legs facing me. His head was about six inches from my crotch and four inches from the recorder I had strapped to the inside of my thigh.

After a while, even some of those who were supposed to be on our side began tracking us. The bureaucrats, tired of being embarrassed, tried to anticipate our next investigation. Looking to cut their losses, they ginned up phoney reports, and launched pre-emptive strikes. Generally, about a week before we were to go to hearing on an issue we had been investigating for a year or more, they'd give up some poor soul who would claim the department already knew about the problem and had it solved.

The act was political, but not partisan. Through the years the administrations of both parties tried to minimize the problem. They questioned and denied first the fact, then the degree of fraud, waste, and abuse. They have been ably assisted in this regard by the American Medical Association, which deserves high marks for consistency.

If our incremental actions have provoked a response of this nature, it is probably unreasonable to expect full disclosure will be more quietly received. When you rattle someone's dish, you can't expect them to sit quietly by or look kindly on you.

Obviously, the possibility of a heated reaction has not proven to be a deterrent. But it does extend the author's obligation to provide a context for the observations and judgements that follow. None of us is entirely without bias. The least we can do is try and state our prejudices as clearly as we can define them.

The principal bias reflected in the pages that follow is that of an investigator. For more than twenty-five years, my brother, Val, and I were engaged in congressional oversight. We worked for both the Senate and the House of Representatives and were responsible for a continuous examination of our nation's health and social programs. We worked as professional staff, investigators, counsel, special counsel, chief counsel, and staff directors. At one point, we held parallel positions – to my knowledge the only time this has occurred – my brother as Director of Oversight and Counsel for a House committee and I in a comparable position for the Senate.

These specific activities should be placed in the context of a broader congressional experience – fifteen years of predicate – during which we did most of the other things that are done on Capitol Hill. We guarded the subway, delivered the mail, worked as gofers, and supervised the operation of the elevators in the Capitol. Last time I heard, I still hold the record for the most time logged going up and down in the Senate – though recent events suggest that record has been subject to serious challenge.

We also worked as speech writers, fundraisers, and research assistants in congressional and presidential campaigns. We have seen the best and worst of our politicians over the last quarter of a century and can tell you the best are much better than they are commonly perceived. The worst are about as bad as they seem – which is bad enough.

Early on, for example, I remember a somewhat brash young man who insisted he would starve if he didn't get a coffee break within the first hour of his five-hour shift. After repeated calls, he finally caught sight of the relief man, only to be informed there would be a further delay as the break man tended to another party with greater seniority.

"When will you be back?" the young one asked impatiently.

"I don't know. He says he is sick."

"What am I supposed to do? I am starving. Can't you bring me a sandwich?"

"No I can't," the relief man said as he went on his way. "But I tell you what. Mike is right behind me. He'll get you one."

It says something about the elevator operator that I was dumb enough to send Mike Mansfield, then Majority Leader of the Senate, for a BLT. It says something about Mansfield that he went.

The new crop has learned to delegate. There are now about 20,000 staffers covering for the 535 members of Congress. Some members would have an aide go to the bathroom for them if they could figure out how to do it.

Democracy is said to rest on the principle that the people know what they want and deserve what they get. It may or may not be what we want, but what we are getting is a variation of the breed that populate television soap operas and game shows, who – in case you have missed it – are the same people who read you the news every night on television.

When we came to Washington, giants walked the halls of Congress. Paul Douglas was one of them. From Douglas we learned something about accountability and responsibility. It is said, the lawmakers of the Thurians had a curious tradition. Anyone who wished either to abolish a law or establish a new one was asked to present himself to the people with a rope around his neck. Douglas would have understood that.

He believed advocates of a particular policy are responsible for the programs they destroy or put in place – responsible for their operation and effectiveness, responsible for the burden they place on the population that supports the program, responsible for the needs unmet.

When we began, the committees were controlled by Democrats. We were frequently reminded at that time that the social programs we were investigating were "democratic" programs. When the issue came up, we remembered Douglas.

Later when the Republicans were in charge of the Executive Branch and still later the committee, the same resistance was raised, following the prevailing Washington wisdom best expressed by Lyndon Johnson, "They may be be SOBs but they are our SOBs." Douglas still applied.

The perspective demanded by the positions we occupied was that of public interest. We were charged with the responsibility of overseeing the operation of hundreds of federal and state programs. Visualize an efficiency expert working for the government, if you can believe such an unlikely combination possible, and you won't be far from the mark.

We were responsible for identifying and eliminating the fraud, waste, and abuse (FAW to the bureaucrats) in programs that account for a third of the federal budget. If you read what follows, you will find we were quite successful in identifying FAW. We were less successful in eliminating it. The why has something to do with this book.

It is often said that we have the best medical system in the world. That may be true if the judgement is seasoned with an America's traditional respect for size, technology, and money.

We spend 12 percent of our GNP on health care – more than $2 billion a day – more than any other country in the world. Yet, at least a dozen countries have greater life expectancy rates for men. Six of these nations also have a greater life expectancy rate for women and most of the developed countries are better at controlling infant mortality.

It is not that our health system is ineffective. In some areas, the progress of medical science is truly startling, and we set the standard for the world. But our system is also monumentally inefficient, progressively wasteful, and increasingly corrupt.

If you were to run an adding tape alongside the incidents described in the chapters that follow, you would find unnecessary and fraudulent health expenditures approaching $60 billion. Like Senator Everett Dirksen used to say, "A million here and a million there and pretty soon you are talking about real money."

Staggering as the total is, it is only a portion of the waste we have documented and only a fraction of the total lost to fraud, waste, and abuse in the last twenty years. If you were to extend and combine the estimates of total loss through the years, you would get a FAW factor of at least 20 percent and as much as 50 percent of total public expenditures. Quite simply, the basic problem is that there isn't enough health in our health care system.

While this waste and our apparent inability to control it appalls me, it is not the sole reason for writing this book. We have enough experience with other branches of the government to know that some of the same problems are present throughout government. Take a look at HUD if you doubt it.

Most troubling is the fact that while we struggle with staggering deficits, which force difficult choices, waste is ignored. Not that it is a secret. Many people, including some politicians, know the problem exists. Some of these politicians, including several presidents, have been elected at least in part because they said they would do something about it.

Yet the problems persist. Instead, we are visited with the wholesale destruction of programs and the mindlessness of universal cuts and caps designed to meet deficit reduction targets. We are asked to choose between expenditures designed to preserve society and programs designed to assure that we have a society worth preserving – as if these were the only choices.

Congress and the administration have embraced "freezes," Gramm-Rudman cuts, and other mechanisms designed to pare down all expenditures, without judgement or distinction between what works and what does not. Meanwhile, our society grows ever more impoverished. Our literacy rate is a scandal. Our health suffers and the homeless fill the streets of our cities.

The implicit message is that we have lost the ability to provide the services our society needs, manage programs, and make intelligent choices. This is a philosophy we firmly reject.

While we will focus in what follows on the problem, please recognize there is at least one hero for every heel, contrary to popular perception. Heros are only less visible. Public servants are the ones who know there is an interest greater than the combination of constituencies with a voice. I learned that from former Senator Frank E. Moss. From the beginning, he would not be bought. He stayed with his convictions even though it cost him party favor and public support. He was and is a man of complete integrity.

From time to time during our congressional careers, we used to muse about the characteristics of a perfect chairman. If you had gathered our notes and built a model based on their design, it would have looked a lot like John Heinz. A man of surpassing intellect, he was able to assimilate months of work in minutes, mastering minutiae as well as he understood the essence. Aggressive and fearless as he was bright, Heinz was the "tiger" we always wanted to press the attack. His only handicap was the natural suspicion with which the establishment greets anyone who is already a millionaire when they arrive in Washington.

The late Claude Pepper managed to distill the essence of public service for me into three words: "Make things better." Over the last fifty years, he did more to make things better than any man I know. Pepper was what I thought they all were when I came to Washington. My only regret is that we didn't find a way to have him declared a national treasure before he died. He should have been put on the "must see" list for every school kid who came to town. He was the most consistently kind and gentle man in Washington.

Others too numerous to mention deserve recognition and thanks. Some of them are: Kathy Gardner who has proven you can do it all; David Holton, who saved my backside more times than I can to mention; Peter Reineke, who was born wiser than most people ever become; Melanie Modlin, who cares as much as anyone can; Marian Brown, who helped prepare this book and refine my thoughts; Joe Hynes, Sam Skinner, and George Wilson, who have managed to restore some of my faith in the judicial system; Bob Eifert, Felix Brunner, and half of the Postal Service's Investigative Unit, who remind me bureaucrat does not have to be a bad word; and Steve Ross, Stan Brand, and John Fine, the three men I would most want with me if I were storming a machine gun nest – come to think of it, they were.

Though I am now out of the government and trying to lead an honorable life, I must confess one final potential conflict of interest. I am still on the dole as a consultant to a house committee.

You've heard of high-priced Washington consultants. I'm paid a dollar a month. I'm one of the few people on the public payroll who can honestly say he is worth every dime he gets.

Chapter One
The Czar of Misery
———❦———

"Where's Scarfone?"

"Who?"

The hospital had three entrances: a public entrance in front, an emergency entrance spiraling out of the parking lot on the north side, and a service entrance in the back. I had come in the back entrance, walked up the stairs and proceeded directly to room 714. I hadn't bothered to ask permission.

I had called the hospital from the airport when I arrived in Miami. Thumbing through the yellow pages, I found the name of a florist I thought vague and innocuous enough.

"This is Tom Kelly with Bayside Florist," I said to the telephone operator. "We have a delivery for Mr. Rocco Scarfone. Can you tell me which room he is in?"

I waited for what seemed a long time for an answer. A six-four, two hundred and forty-pound patient in traction shouldn't be all that hard to find.

Finally, I heard a vague conversation in the background as the operator discussed the matter with someone. A moment later, she came back on the line. She said, "He's in 714."

The man I found in 714 was about my height and age. He looked to be about as healthy, except for the cast on his left leg.

"Skiing," he said.

In addition to being bigger and older, the man I was looking for from all descriptions was near death's door. You pretty much have to be if you are going to avoid a Senate subpoena.

First we were told Rocco had prostate problems that required surgery. Then he had rheumatoid arthritis and a bad disc. Finally, we were told he had to be placed in traction and could not be moved for an indefinite period.

When we pressed the issue, his physician became testy and told us Rocco had all of the above. Not only would he require prostate surgery, but he would also need surgery to repair damaged discs in his spinal column. In the interim, he had also developed emphysema and arteriosclerosis.

Scarfone couldn't travel. He couldn't talk. He couldn't move. He couldn't have visitors. He would not be able to appear before the Senate committee or give a deposition. This side of Lourdes, he wouldn't have been able to go skiing.

I went looking for the nurses' station and found a friendly young woman behind the counter. She offered me a slice of the melon she had brought for lunch. "He checked out this morning," she said.

"Oh?"

I had another slice of melon.

"How is he feeling?"

"He's all right. He's in and out of here all the time."

The committee was investigating the operation of nursing homes. The focus of our investigation was Rabbi Bernard Bergman. Bergman was said to have stolen millions of dollars from medicaid.

He had come to the United States as a teenager in 1929. Three years later he had begun his career as a chaplain in a nursing home on New York's east side. Though he would deny it, our investigations indicated he now had interests in at least sixty nursing homes across the country.

He was then sixty-three and a multi-millionaire. He was said to be a "fine gentleman" by some and a "merchant of misery" by others. There was no dispute about his position in the community, or about his power. He had contributed heavily to both political parties for years and was known to be well-connected.

He was a significant supporter of President Nixon and then Governor Nelson Rockefeller. He was on intimate terms with the Speaker of the New York Assembly, Stanley Steingut, and the Brooklyn Democratic boss Meade H. Esposito.

He was well enough thought of that he was even allowed to open a session of the House of Representatives, saying a prayer and asking God to guide the deliberations of the body. At about the same time Bergman's father, Rabbi Leifer, was arrested in France for trying to smuggle heroin into the United States. He had concealed the drugs in compartments cut out of prayer books.

When arrested, Leifer's defense was that he was a famous American rabbi. The dope was merely sand, he said, from the Holy Land. He was convicted in France, sentenced to two years in prison, and then extradited to the United States.

John Hess, a first-rate reporter with the *New York Times* had kicked open the Bergman investigation. Hess had determined that most of New York's nursing homes were owned by a few people. He found a wide pattern of poor care, patient abuse, and profiteering.

The committee, with my brother Val's guidance, had just completed a landmark three-year investigation of nursing homes in the United States. The committee's national findings mirrored Hess' New York experience. The committee concluded that more than half of the nursing homes in the United States were substandard and presented life-threatening conditions.

In an unprecedented move, then Congressman Ed Koch asked the committee to investigate Hess' allegations. No one on the state level had broad enough jurisdiction. No one else on the federal level had the committee's experience.

The committee agreed. Within two weeks, Val had reviewed the surface documents and responded with characteristic caution. He subpoenaed everything and everyone remotely connected with the case. More than sixty subpoenas were executed in all. Each one touched a nerve and triggered calls to flocks of high-priced New York lawyers.

Not to worry, Val said, we had them outnumbered. After all, there were two of us.

A preliminary investigation by the General Accounting Office requested by Val for the committee immediately confirmed the substance of Hess' allegations. Over a million dollars was said to be missing from the account of one of Bergman's nursing homes. Another $2.2 million had been paid out of the home's account to Bergman and his relatives.

Almost as quickly, another thread of the investigation led to the mob. One of Bergman's partners, Samuel Klurman, had a somewhat checkered past. The Pinkerton report we obtained indicated some thirteen court actions against him in a five-year period.

One of Klurman's associates, Joseph Cannistracci, had recently disappeared under gaudy circumstances. Word was someone had put six bullets through him and rolled him into the East River shortly before he was to appear at a congressional hearing. He was now said to be underground and unavailable for comment.

And then there were the ties to Joe Columbo. The notorious mob figure seemed to permeate the atmosphere of the investigation. Our best direct connection was Rocco Scarfone.

Bergman was said to be laundering money in the Bahamas. An informer inside the operation fingered Rocco as the runner. As evidence she repeated a conversation she had overheard. Rocco had called one of the airlines in great distress. It seemed the airline had lost his baggage. But Rocco only seemed concerned about the loss of one small package. The package bore Bergman's name.

The airline based in Florida confirmed the incident. We also had confirmation that Rocco was a frequent visitor to and part-time resident of Bergman's Park Central penthouse – an intriguing lifestyle for a former New York City cop.

The administrator of the Miami hospital was a small nervous man. He had kept me waiting for the better part of an hour. Fortunately, I'd had lunch.

He made a point of examining my credentials. While he jotted down my name I asked him where Rocco was.

"I don't know," he said.

"How long has he been gone?"

"I don't know," he said.

"When did you find out he was gone?"

"I just now found out."

"How long was he here?"

"I don't know."

"Why was he admitted?"

"I can't tell you." He seemed to be getting more nervous by the minute. "That's privileged information."

Sometimes I appear a little too intense. I smiled and tried to look amiable. "That's not exactly true. There are at least two ways you can tell me. One is if I make a call to the chairman and he sends the federal marshals down here with subpoena for your records – all of your records. The other is with permission. Which would you prefer?"

The administrator said he would seek permission. He started to call Rocco's physician, thought better of it, and put down the phone. "The matter is difficult," he said. "The physician is not a member of the hospital."

"How is it he has privileges?"

"It's a special case," the administrator said.

I asked if he thought highly of the physician and the administrator seemed relieved. Finally, I had given him a question he could answer.

"Let's put it this way," he said, "if my daughter was sick, I would tell her to go to someone else."

"Does he have a specialty?"

"He's a cardiologist."

It seemed to be a strange way to go after a prostate problem. I wanted to ask the doctor about that, but he was nowhere to be found. His office said he was on vacation.

But within an hour of my visit, he called the committee. "I don't know who in the hell you think you guys are," he told Val, "or who you think you're dealing with, but if you push us around we are going to push back."

Val said he had a flat, nasal voice, and a peculiar almost Australian accent. Val said since the man seemed to be so unhappy, he had sent the marshals with a couple of pieces of paper to cheer him up. The committee also issued subpoenas for Rocco and his medical records. In light of Rocco's delicate condition, we arranged transportation and an escort to the hearing.

The committee found Bergman and company were taking the taxpayers for a ride. Nursing homes owned by Bergman and his friends were "churned" – sold back and forth to related parties in order to inflate their equity. One facility had been sold and resold thirty-four times, the first time for $250,000 and the last time for $5.7 million. The public picked up tab for each transaction.

Alternatively, one of the nursing homes would be sold and then leased back, allowing the seller to deduct the expenses associated with paying rent and still profit from the sale. Meanwhile, the books of the nursing homes were being manipulated to show a loss. On average their assets were about one tenth their liabilities.

The books of one of two dozen homes investigated showed paper losses of $1.1 million over six years. When we backed out the excessive rent the owners paid themselves, the home showed a profit of $840,000 and that did not include the hundreds of thousands of dollars paid out in salaries to partners, wives, and families.

It was part of what was already a familiar pattern. The federal health programs enacted in the mid-60s were the result of five decades of debate. National health insurance programs were proposed by presidents Theodore Roosevelt in 1912, Franklin Roosevelt in 1944, Harry Truman in 1945, John Kennedy in 1960, and Lyndon Johnson in 1965.

Though the initial response of the medical community was favorable – in 1915 the American Medical Association advertised it was putting the final touches on a model health insurance program – the support soon evaporated. In 1920 the AMA retrenched, stating unqualified opposition to any form of health insurance controlled or regulated in any way by the state or federal government.

The balance turned during the presidential election of 1960. Kennedy made health insurance a principal part of his campaign and Nixon responded. But one critical compromise had already been made: both candidates were talking about health insurance programs offering partial coverage with eligibility restricted by age and income.

In the five years that remained before enactment of medicare and medicaid, further compromises were made. All of them came back to haunt us. Many haunt us still.

One of these was the disagreement as to whether the state government or the federal government should run the new program. Either option would have been preferable in the long run to the compromise that divided authority and responsibility.

The other compromise was even more costly. The purpose of medicare and medicaid was to make "mainstream medicine" available to those who couldn't afford to pay for it themselves. Doctors were paid their "customary" fee, whatever that was or whatever they wanted it to be. In both cases, payment was made virtually without review.

To perfect the disaster, we agreed to insulate the medical community from the disgrace of receiving money directly from the government. It was agreed the possibility of contamination would be camouflaged by passing it through intermediaries created and controlled by hospitals and physicians. In short, the medical community asked for and received a blank check as their condition of participation.

It should not have been a surprise that within a year of the program's initiation, the government had to increase medicare taxes by 25 percent in order to meet the unexpectedly high costs of the program. Within five years, there was evidence that the medicare and medicaid programs were in serious difficulty. Costs were running about twice what they had been expected to be.

The committee had been instrumental in the development of medicare and medicaid. Much of the final impetus for the legislation had been supplied by a series of national hearings begun in 1959 which ran through 1960. The committee had found that despite the fact that health costs of seniors were twice that of the young, only half of the elderly had hospital insurance. Less than half were insured against the cost of surgical procedures.

Now, less than ten years after the program had begun, we were facing mounting evidence that the long-term viability of the program was in jeopardy. Inescapably, the purposes of the program were being perverted by the profit motive and greed of a few unscrupulous people.

When Rocco was served, he threw the subpoena back in the marshal's face. He none the less appeared before the committee two weeks later. He was a great, suntanned, hulk of a man. He looked about as decrepit as pier piling.

"My name is Rocco, R-O-C-C-0. The middle initial is A. The last name is Scarfone. S-C-A-R-F-O-N-E," he said like a man accustomed to the circumstances.

He was asked if he were hospitalized at the time he had declined the committee's previous invitation.

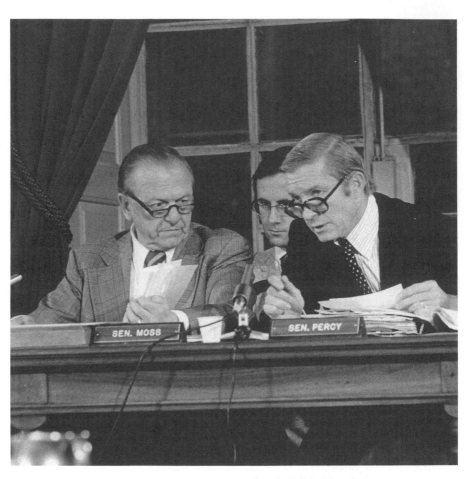

photo by Bill Halamandaris
Senators Moss and Percy during the Bergman hearing.

Rocco pointed to the soft whiplash collar around his neck and said he was.

"Did you have any medical procedure while you were there?"

"Yes."

"What was that procedure?"

"I was anaesthetized."

"For what reason?"

"For my prostate and a vasectomy, which was not completed."

When asked if he had ever been employed by Bergman, Scarfone at first denied any such relationship, then recanted on cross-examination, saying he had misunderstood the question.

The committee had documented laundry services as one of the most common connections between nursing homes and the mob. Rocco admitted he first met Bergman while working for Star Laundry. He said he was investigating the theft of linens in the homes.

"Who owns the linen company?" Senator Percy asked.

"I don't know."

"In Chicago it is reasonably well known that certain legitimate businesses have been taken over by the syndicate. They have fronts. That's their way of doing business and I'm sure I don't have to explain that to you. So, I ask you specifically, who owns this linen company?"

"I don't know."

"Who did you work for?"

"Saudi Goldberg."

"How did it happen that this particular linen company was interested in doing business with nursing homes?"

"I don't know."

"How did it happen that Dr. Bergman hired you and paid you thousands of dollars to presumably investigate the theft of linens in his nursing homes?"

Scarfone explained he had come to know Bergman in the course of his duties as a salesman for the laundry service. He said they had become friends.

"I'm sorry," Percy concluded, "that just doesn't wash."

Under cross-examination, Rocco admitted Bergman had given him a personal loan to start a private detective agency and paid him thousands of dollars for security work.

He admitted frequent trips between Miami and New York and confirmed the telephone conversation reported by our informant. He also admitted he knew Joe Columbo. Though he was close to Columbo and called him friend, Rocco said their relationship was limited to matters affecting Italian-American civil rights.

"What did you call him and what did he call you?" he was asked.

"I called him Joseph," Scarfone said, "and he called me Rocco."

Following the investigation, Bergman plead guilty to fraud. He was sentenced to one year in jail and ordered to repay $2.5 million plus 8 percent interest.

Rocco took a walk.

His physician declined our invitation to appear before the committee. The committee felt we didn't have enough evidence to compel his appearance.

Chapter Two
Chercher La Buck

Wallace was surprised. Abandoning his observation point, he had come out from behind the one-way glass to confront the salesman.

"I'm Mike Wallace with CBS 'Sixty Minutes,'" he said quickly. "Did I just hear you offer this man a kickback?"

Wallace had expected fear, denial, or panic, perhaps something akin to cardiac arrest. Instead the salesman barely broke stride. He nodded his head and went on with his pitch.

Maybe he doesn't recognize you, someone suggested. Wallace's reply was short and emphatic. It was early 1975. We were in Chicago on an educational mission. Governor Daniel Walker had expressed the public belief that there wasn't any fraud in Illinois. We thought he was confused and that it might help if we showed him what it looked like.

Six months earlier in sworn testimony, John Goff, a former state employee, had blamed the administration for wasting at least $350 million of the taxpayers' money. "The major reason why this waste has continued in Illinois," he said, "is the direct interjection of politics into the management and administrative processes of the welfare department."

The governor was on the phone in the back of the hearing room screaming his displeasure before Goff had finished the first page of testimony. "What in the f— do you think you are doing down there?" he asked. Even though he had been briefed earlier as to the nature of Goff's testimony in a courtesy call, he still sounded surprised. "You can't put that nut on the stand! He's a zealot."

Until a few months before the hearing, Goff had been the section chief for the state's Department of Quality Control. In that position, he had been responsible for supervising 200 employees. A computer whiz, he was among those appointed by the man who now called him a nut to a blue ribbon panel, which was supposed to clean up the state's medicaid program.

While the governor fumed, Goff testified he had been instructed not to cancel more than 3,000 ineligible welfare cases a week before the state's primary elections in 1974.

"Stop this hearing," the governor demanded. "What kind of Democrats do you have down there? You're being used by the Republicans to hurt me."

Goff testified there had been repeated attempts to recruit people working the federally funded programs to work in the governor's campaign.

"I created a task force to clean this up," the governor said.

Goff testified the task force was a sham. The whole thing was a farce, he said, a public relations maneuver.

"I can't believe I'm getting stuck with this," Governor Walker said. "Why don't you dig around and see who put him up to this?"

"Goff's been vouched for by the state's attorney general, the comptroller's office, and George Bliss, among others."

"They're all Republicans, aren't they?"

"I didn't know Bliss was. I always thought he was a pretty good reporter."

"That's just as bad. The *Tribune* is always on my back."

Goff testified he had been instructed not to cooperate with federal investigators trying to determine the amount of waste in Illinois in the hopes "they would get discouraged and simply go away."

"I can't believe you did this without checking with me first," the governor said.

"We checked the facts rather thoroughly, Governor. There's a lot of fraud and waste up there and not much evidence the state has done anything to clean it up."

"That's not true. I've made it one of the priorities of my administration."

In contrast to the governor's heated denials, Goff spoke flatly without emotion. "Money is being diverted from the purpose for which it was appropriated," he said, looking like the stereotype of the accountant he was. "Tens of millions are being ripped off by medical vendors who are engaged in wholesale fraud and the State of Illinois has responded by sweeping it under the rug."

That afternoon, in a hastily called press conference, the governor responded for the record. He said Goff "lied" and called the committee staff "irresponsible." He also contacted one of the senior Democrats on the committee, Lawton Chiles, a friend from another life. Chiles listened with the sympathetic ear of a friend and then took us to the woodshed in open session. The senator expressed his concern for the committee's conduct, suggesting it was inappropriate for the committee to be playing "gotcha."

It was the first and only time we were blind-sided. From that point forward, we began every investigation by examining the connections of the subjects to members of Congress, anticipating and sealing off opposition. After a while, we were able to identify the members by whose pocket they were in. Some of them are in more pockets than lint.

Clearly, the governor took it personally. I have to admit, so did we.

By this time we had conducted more than two dozen investigations of problems in the medicare and medicaid programs. We had seen doctors who removed warts and charged for the removal of "cancerous lesions." We'd seen doctors who walked through nursing homes once a month file claims for visits to every patient in the facility. We'd seen patients who went to clinics for ear piercing wind up with bills for hundreds of dollars in lab tests.

A Michigan man had charged the government over $700 for lab tests related to a simple rash. A Chicago teenager was given twenty-six pairs of eyeglasses – all useless – at taxpayer expense. Each time he complained, he was given a new pair at government expense.

We'd found cases where the same bills were submitted and paid two and three times in a period of a month, and providers who charged liquor and imported cigars, travel to the Nixon inaugural, and an orchestra for a lavish Christmas party to the government as a medical expense.

When questioned, party's host admitted the offense but explained, "It wasn't much of an orchestra."

One of his competitors, a former employee, billed the government for oil paintings, jewelry, a Mercedes, clothing, and a motor home for her dog who was afraid to fly. In addition, taxpayers were asked to subsidize the operation of her beauty salon, support her sister, daughter, and son-in-law in style, and pay off the man who was charged by the government with the responsibility of auditing her accounts. In a rare display of chutzpa, she gave him a $14,000 sports car and charged this bribe, like everything else, to Uncle Sam.

In Colorado, Arden Bridge had told us about his career as "the number one head hunter in Colorado." A small, nervous man, this convicted felon had lied about his past and was given a license to operate a nursing home. Bridge bragged he could pull patients out of the trees, running his nursing home at 120 percent occupancy. People were put up in cots in halls, closets, and in the attic.

When the word of his success spread, people began offering him up to eighty dollars a head to find patients for them. It didn't matter if occasionally the patients were dead. The body was brought in by ambulance, logged in, given a bed for a few minutes, and sent on to the morgue. Meanwhile, forms were forged to indicate the patient had died shortly after entering the nursing home.

In one of our most extensive investigations, we reviewed 100 reports issued during the first ten years of the medicaid program. Some $3 billion was said to have been wasted in New York alone during that period due to fraud and abuse. One of the reports, a 1972 grand jury report, concluded that half of the $2 billion New York City had spent on medicaid from 1966 to 1969 had been wasted.

Among the abuses identified in a 1,500 page grand jury report was the story of a dentist who was found to have drilled holes in healthy teeth to create cavities, or rather, evidence of cavities, which justified fillings that could be billed to the government. Another dentist was found to have removed six teeth from a seven-year old's mouth on six different occasions, spreading out the procedures just because he received an extra ten dollars each time he administered the anaesthesia. Podiatrists were found to be x-raying the feet of every patient they saw, and billing the paring of corns as a surgical procedure.

Judge Jacob Grumet had presided over the New York Grand Jury. He had just retired when we met, but he remembered the case. "I handled a lot of cases," he said. "Maybe you don't remember them all, but $1 billion is a lot to forget." He said the doctors were routinely billing for services they hadn't provided, adding, "I've never seen an instance where the city has allowed itself to be so easily fleeced."

In Chicago, a dozen inner-city pharmacies were found to be forging prescriptions, inflating the bills by more than a thousand percent. Nursing homes ordered ten-day supplies of drugs every two to three days, with the overage going to the streets. Hospital employees were bribed to deliver bodies to funeral homes or asked to double as runners, alerting the funeral home of the death of terminal patients before the families were notified. One witness graphically described for us the runners "hovering over patients and waiting for them to die" like the vultures they were.

We estimated that 10 percent of the $30 billion being spent at that time for medicare and medicaid was either wasted or stolen, with the worst fraud occurring in the medicaid program. Both the states and the federal government are responsible for policing medicaid. The theory is that both have interests to protect and that two is better than one. In practice, the result is reminiscent of Abbot and Costello baseball: "I've got it, you take it."

A quarter of the states had not prosecuted a single case of medicaid fraud in the first ten years of the program. Twenty-one states had not even bothered to audit a single provider of services.

The fed's response was equally distressing. The Department of Health, Education and Welfare counted medicare and medicaid as only two of the 334 programs they were responsible for administering even though these two programs tallied about a third of the federal budget. Medicare and medicaid listed a combined total of 140,000 employees. Twenty-three of them were said to be investigators.

Given the odds, it should not have been a surprise the con men and crooks were having such a field day. Each year of the program brought a progressive increase in the size and nature of the rip-off schemes. In one survey we did of pharmacies doing business with the government, 63 percent of the 2,000 people we asked admitted to being involved in kickback schemes or other illegal activities. They placed the average kickback at about 25 percent. They admitted bribing their customers at taxpayers' expense with everything from cash to cars, mink coats, jewelry, and travel to exotic places. Meanwhile, ethical providers were losing money. Charles Brown, President of the California Pharmaceutical Association, blasted the corrupt practices saying he personally had lost over $200,000 in business just because he wouldn't play the game.

When we asked the General Accounting Office to determine how many nursing homes were stealing from their patients, they audited homes in six states and came back with the first 100 percent sample I had ever seen. Every home surveyed was found guilty of stealing the small living allowance Congress provided for the personal use of nursing home residents.

Administration of the medicaid program was in such disarray, middlemen called factoring firms were making fortunes by promising the medical community prompt payment. The disorganization was so total and the profit so enormous, some questioned the coincidence. A number of the key players in these schemes, which came to resemble legalized loan sharking, were tied to the underworld.

A physician in Illinois told us how he came to regret his association with the factoring firms. Seduced by the promise of prompt payment and frustrated by the government's inefficiency, he had signed on, promising the factors 12 percent of the value of each bill for cash up front. Only later did he figure out that 12 percent annually was not the same as 12 percent monthly. He was also surprised to find that the bills the factor submitted and were reimbursed for in his name were significantly larger than the bills he had initially submitted.

In June of 1974, Dr. Caroll Hutchinson, then President of the Cook County Medical Association, took the matter to the press. He complained the Illinois Department of Public Aid was cooperating in "a multi-million dollar rip-off racket." The state has encouraged the development of these middlemen, he said, when it was obvious it was a racket.

"Factoring has the same odious characteristics as the juice racket," Hutchinson charged, noting factors were somehow able to collect payment from the state immediately, while providers would sometimes have to wait as long as two years for payment of the same claim.

Goff confirmed Hutchinson's allegations. He said the department's records showed only eleven factoring firms in Illinois. But his computer analysis had found more than thirty in operation. Further, his analysis documented the fact that factors were paid more promptly. They were also found to have submitted an extraordinary number of bills that were marked with an override code designed to bypass all computer checks and validations. One of these factors was said to have made about $10 million in two years. They also kited about half of the 4,000 invoices we examined.

In August, a member of the Illinois medical payments section admitted taking cash and gifts for providing confidential information and expediting payment to the factoring companies. A month later, a past president of the Chicago Medical Society issued a scathing report on behalf of the state's Medical Advisory Committee. His report criticized the "assembly-line" treatment of patients, bill-padding, and poor care. Some doctors were said to billing for 100 to 150 patients a day – or one patient every three minutes. Most of the doctors were said to bc foreign medical school graduates. Some of them were said to be relying on unlicensed people to make their diagnoses and provide care.

In December, the state's attorney general added to the litany of abuses, charging the Department of Public Aid had been sitting on evidence of massive fraud by a group of pharmacies for more than a year. They reported "incredible evidence of wholesale fraud" so obvious it was visible to the naked eye. Additions were made in handwriting visibly different from the physicians' and in an ink of a different color.

When confronted, the Department of Public Aid at first denied having the evidence and then reported the files were missing. The state's attorney had to spend weeks forcing the state Welfare Department to surrender the evidence.

Then there was Ed Morgan.

Ed Morgan was the Executive Secretary of the Illinois Clinical Laboratory Association. A meek man with a pencil moustache, Morgan called the committee to say how "distressed" he was about the practices of unethical laboratory facilities. "Criminal elements have purchased many of the laboratories," he said. They were performing "sink tests" (pouring the specimen down the sink and billing as if they'd been tested), submitting phoney bills, and padding invoices.

Morgan said the labs routinely paid off the doctors. Doctors were given a percentage of the money the government paid for the tests as an inducement to do

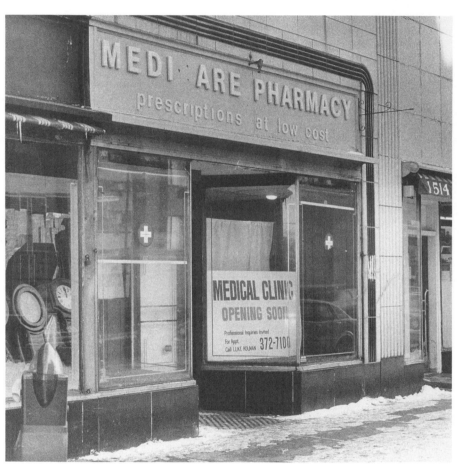

The clinic on Morris Avenue.

photo by Bill Halamandaris

business. When we asked him how much, he said that one out of every six medicaid dollars paid for lab tests was being ripped off.

Morgan said he had presented his evidence to the governor's task force. The governor said he had cleaned it up. Goff said they were covering it up. We said we'd see.

That led to the creation of the clinic on Morris Avenue where Mike Wallace engaged Bill Minor, the business manager of Northside Laboratories in a frank discussion. By this time, Walter Dumbro, CBS' cameraman had also come around from behind the mirror.

"It's a fact of life," Minor said. "In the inner city, that's the way it's done."

"And you know who picks up the tab. The taxpayer."

"We'd be out of business tomorrow," Minor said. "It's as simple as that."

"If you weren't kicking back to the doctors?"

"Right."

In the wake of Goff's testimony and Morgan's appearance before the committee, we had been contacted by Dr. Herbert Meyer. He said he had been approached by Westlawn Laboratory. Meyer wanted to know if he would be in trouble if he took their offer. We said we'd send someone up to help.

On October 14, 1975 our consultant sat in Meyer's closet and heard Westlawn's salesman go over their "incentive plan."

"It's 30 percent," the salesman said.

"How do you handle it?"

"There are a number of ways. We can pay rent, help cover your overhead, or give you cash."

"Well, anything I get goes on the books," Meyer said.

"Don't worry. There are loopholes in every law. We do this with doctors and clinics all over town." He went on to explain that the laboratory had similar arrangements with six clinics and dozens of individual physicians.

That's when we decided to open our own clinic. We rented a storefront on the south side, put a sign in the window, and made a few calls. We said we were a couple of young physicians opening up for business. From there, we just sat back and let it roll. For three weeks, lab representatives streamed through the door. The people we saw controlled 70 percent of the medicaid business in the state. All but two offered us a deal.

William Footlick was one of the players. The owner of the lab doing the largest volume of public aid business in the state, he laid it out. He offered "a percentage of the volume of public aid business you do."

"How much?"

"Twenty-five to 30 percent."

"Is that rental for space or what?"

"A rose is a rose."

"How much space would the lab need?"

"A blood drawer, a chair, and a cabinet. For that you ought to average $5,000 to $6,000 a month." Rent for the entire storefront was $450 a month.

Footlick's competitors offered kickbacks ranging from 25 to 50 percent. The best offer came from Division. They said they'd kick back 30 percent of our

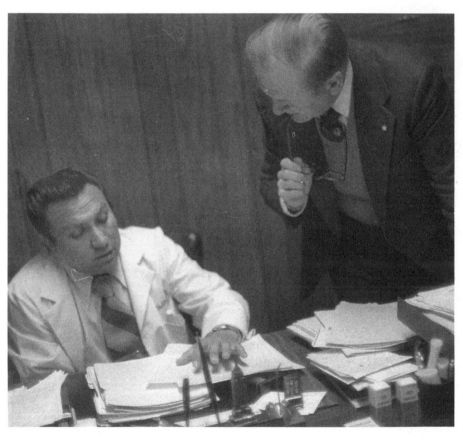

photo by Val Halamandaris

"I didn't order these."
Dr. Lara-Valle with Senator Moss.

gross, pick up the salary of one of our employees, plus the cost of equipment and supplies, x-ray technicians' services, and provide electrical and plumbing services for the clinic. Whether the space they "rented" was used or not seemed immaterial. "We just need a foot or so for the IRS," one salesman said candidly, "just to make it look legal."

"Sixty Minutes" entered the picture in October when Marion Golden called looking for input on another story. In the process, Val told her what we were up to. By December we knew what we had and they wanted a piece of it. While Wallace and company conducted their interviews, we extended our findings. We had direct information from the labs. We decided to take it the next step and confront the physicians with whom they worked.

Armed with hundreds of paid invoices, we walked into four dozen clinics and confronted the doctors who worked there. In every case, the physician confirmed the kickback arrangement. Some extended it.

Dr. Julio Lara-Valle was one of these. He was a short, pudgy man. He wore his hair slicked back in a pompadour. His mouth twitched nervously when I asked him how much he had received from the laboratory.

"A thousand dollars a month," he said finally.

"How much do you pay in rent for the entire office?"

"Three hundred dollars."

"Does the lab provide any other services?"

"They also give me another thousand for rent for the pharmacy next door."

His nervousness shifted to apoplexy when I asked him to review the invoices submitted in his name. He kept shaking his head, saying "I didn't order these." Each bill had been padded. The laboratory had increased the number of tests ordered in our sample by 55 percent.

When we reviewed the premises occupied by the labs, we found most did not begin to have the capacity to perform the volume of tests they had billed. In one case, we found samples waiting in a beer cooler for pickup. In another, a routine blood count was waiting for pickup by another lab for analysis. The sample belonged to the owner's wife. At a third facility, we opened a refrigerator to find blood samples, stools, and other specimens sharing space with the technician's lunch.

Meanwhile, a comparison tour of a nearby multi-million dollar automated facility run by the Masonic Hospital revealed more hardware than all the other labs combined. There were rows upon rows of sophisticated equipment.

"How much medicaid business does this lab do?" we asked the director.

"Very little," he said. They refused to take kickbacks.

Our findings in Illinois were replicated in other states. The General Accounting Office reported that three-fifths of the doctors they reviewed for us in four states were adding markups of 100 to 400 percent to the lab charges. The fact that the American Medical Association had resolved that "any markup, commission, or profit" by doctors on outside lab tests amounts to "exploitation of the patient" seemed to matter no more than the question of its legality.

In New York we found that sixteen clinical laboratories controlled 70 percent of the medicaid business. In New Jersey, a dozen clinics controlled more than 60

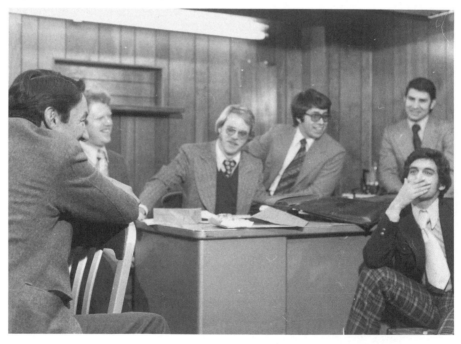

photo by Val Halamandaris
Mike Wallace with investigators inside the clinic on Morris Avenue.

percent of the business. In both states, just as we'd seen in Illinois, labs that didn't play the kickback game were closed out.

The chairman of the board of MetPath Labs, Inc., one of the largest testing firms in the country, said that less than $10,000 of the company's $2 million in annual billings came from medicaid. The reason, he said, was the firm's decision to obey the law and avoid kickback arrangements.

We concluded the government was losing a minimum of $45 million of the $213 million it was then paying for laboratory services to medicare and medicaid patients. We guessed the total loss, based on the kickbacks we were offered, was probably closer to one dollar out of every five.

If you add the dollars lost as a result of kited fee schedules and padded bills, the loss was even greater. The best estimate of total loss was provided by the State of New York. Faced with this mess, the state decided to establish a competitive bidding process for all the state's medicaid business. They concluded they could provide the same service at half the cost.

The findings of our investigation of clinical labs were released on February 16, 1976. CBS had gone with their story the night before. On February 17, the State of Illinois suspended four clinical laboratories. The *Chicago Tribune* quoted Joel Edelman, director of a bipartisan investigative committee, as saying his investigators had turned over evidence on the labs in question, in addition to four others more than a year and a half earlier. "For a year or more, there was some kind of cover-up going on," Edelman said. "Now that there is some heat on, a lot of this stuff is finally starting to come out into the open."

Governor Walker announced the appointment of fifty new medicaid fraud investigators. He seemed to have gotten the message, but lost his re-election bid none the less. The owner of one of the labs we'd investigated went off the bridge. Another disappeared from sight and has not been seen since.

As a reward for cooperating with the committee, Dr. Meyer's life was threatened. His car was vandalized. His practice suffered and he felt compelled to relocate to another state.

Chapter Three
Everybody's Doing It
—— 🍂 ——

"Anybody have an idea how I can fill this bottle?"

Senator Moss was speaking into a wireless strapped inside his denim jacket.

"I'm sure she won't let me out of here unless I give her something."

The senator was tapped out. Dressed in his World War II khakis, he was making his third stop in the space of a few hours. In each of the clinics, he had been bounced from doctor to doctor, jabbed with needles, diagnosed to be suffering from some unlikely disease or another, and asked to give a specimen.

Outside, in a surveillance van we had borrowed from the IRS, we heard a cabinet open. "Maybe this will do," he said. "It's about the right color and smells foul enough. When you shake it, it even foams." While Moss dressed, the nurse dropped a labstick into the cleaning fluid. She pronounced it normal.

We were in New York at the conclusion of a massive effort designed to test the quality of care being given to the poor and elderly. Over the years, hundreds of witnesses had testified to the fact that there was a relation between fraud, financial abuses, and substandard care. Rarely, was one present without the other. Their testimony was upheld by dozens of instances where we had documented patient abuse and negligence in nursing homes and other settings. However, at this point there was little direct systemic evidence.

The poor and the elderly had been promised they would have access to mainstream medicine; that they would get the same kind of care the rest of us get. It was assumed we had succeeded. But there was enough episodic evidence to the contrary to warrant a hard look.

We decided to test the quality of services the only way possible – by putting ourselves in the positions of the patients, the people the system was designed to serve. We prepared by reviewing the payment records of doctors in the five states that accounted for the majority of the government's health expenditures. We had surveyed some 150 physicians in New York and interviewed some fifty physicians in California, Illinois, New Jersey, Michigan, and New York as to the nature of their priorities.

Friends, Jim Roberts and Scotty McDew, had been borrowed from the Capitol Hill police force. Interns and other staff members were drafted for spot duty. The Physician of the Capitol had been prevailed upon to examine our team and certify our good health.

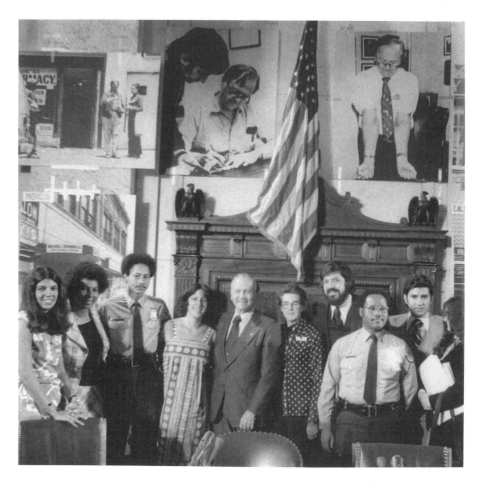

photo by Bill Oriol
Senator Moss with medicaid mills investigative team.

The U.S. Attorney provided blank medicaid cards, which we personalized with whimsical names. My brother was always fond of Lester P. Gilles for some reason. The U.S. Attorney also arranged a tracking mechanism for the bills generated by our rounds.

Armed with these cards and street corner credentials, we presented ourselves for treatment in hundreds of clinics in the five states – New York, New Jersey, Michigan, Illinois, and California. We presented the simplest of complaints – most often, "I think I have a cold."

With that scant excuse, we were subjected to hundreds of x-rays (on average, three per patient per clinic visit), dozens of electrocardiograms, tuberculosis tests, allergy tests, hearing tests, and glaucoma exams. We were treated to three electroencephalograms and given a dozen pair of glasses.

We were "ping-ponged" to neurologists, gynecologists, internists, psychologists, psychiatrists, heart specialists, podiatrists, dentists, chiropractors, opticians, ophthalmologists, optometrists and pediatricians. In some clinics, we literally had to run out of the clinic to end the merry-go-round. Only once did a physician tell any of us, "Get out of here. There's nothing wrong with you."

We formed the firm impression that most of these people wouldn't know how to determine what was wrong with you if something was, nor would they know what to do about it. We also got the impression that they didn't much care.

Despite the severity of many of the diagnoses, most of the doctors did not touch us. Examinations were brief and from a distance. One physician examined my throat by asking me to say "aahh" and shining a flashlight into my mouth from across the room. Temperatures and blood pressures were not taken. Nor did they examine our eyes, ears, or mouths except in a cursory fashion.

In one clinic on the East Side of Manhattan, three of us were diagnosed as having severe "heart murmurs" in the space of thirty minutes. We were all subjected to EKGs and TB tests, given large amounts of medication, and scheduled for follow-up visits.

Scotty walked into a clinic in Harlem with a "head cold" and walked out with ankle braces, a "hammer toe," and an arch support (a rubber cushion) placed in his shoes. In Detroit, I complained of a sore arm. I was diagnosed as being depressed – probably because my pitching days were over. I was given Elavil (an "upper") and Valium (a "downer"), antibiotics, and vitamins. Three times I had to refuse a shot "guaranteed" to make me feel better.

In California, we picked up some medicaid cards that had been forged by inmates at Folsom Prison. Using one, Jim walked into a clinic in Los Angeles and was given an allergy test, chest x-ray, and EKG before seeing a physician. He was scheduled for an ear, nose, and throat examination at a later date.

The bills that came in to justify our "treatment" indicated diagnoses of tyloma (a callus on the foot), severe urinary tract infections, flat feet, insomnia, hay fever, bronchitis, tension, chest pains, cystitis, bilateral hyvalgus, taplipes valgus (club foot), asthma, anxiety, hypertension, conjunctivitis, and in-grown toenails. The treatment of an in-grown toenail was billed as a surgical procedure.

We were not only billed for conditions we did not have, we were billed by doctors we did not see. In at least two dozen cases, bills came in indicating we had been treated in places we hadn't been on days we were somewhere else.

We had allergy and tuberculosis tests that were not read.

We had our chests and feet x-rayed with dental equipment, and x-rays given without plates in the machine or without changing plates. One character x-rayed my feet off a manila envelope claiming it worked just as well and was cheaper. He may have been right.

We had EKGs where the tapes were not marked and dated, and others where the electrodes were placed over clothing.

We saw disposable needles reused and clinics with one thermometer – a rectal at that!

In all of our visits, we never had anything like an adequate medical history taken. In fact, we never spent more than ten minutes with any one physician.

Meanwhile, all around us we saw the ill go unaided. While we waited to be processed, we were surrounded by people with real and serious illnesses – diabetes, severe tachycardia, tuberculosis, syphilis and gonorrhea, rheumatoid arthritis, malnutrition, heart disease, and cancer.

One of the cancer victims wound up seeing a physician who cooperated with us. The patient said he had had a tracheotomy some twelve years earlier and had had recurring pain since that time.

The physician examined the external wound and found it had healed properly. In examining the man further, she asked him to open his mouth and discovered a tumor the size of an egg. He said he had been visiting various clinics in New York seeking relief for more than three years but this was the first time anyone had asked him to open his mouth.

In Illinois we found a clinic that claimed every serology that was performed was positive. The same clinic gave me a hematocrit reading, which, if it were to be believed, would have meant I was hemorrhaging and near death on one day and receiving whole blood transfusions on the next.

A patient we spoke to while waiting in a Bronx clinic indicated he was there because he had syphilis. He knew he had that disease because he had been treated for the same condition before being released from the army. The only treatment he received in three visits to the clinic was provided by a chiropractor.

At our request, a physician examined the records of a patient who had repeatedly sought assistance in a Brooklyn clinic for recurring chest pain. She found the thirty-five-year-old patient had suffered a myocardial infarction (heart attack). The good news was the condition was reflected in the electrocardiogram taken by the clinic. The bad news was that no one had ever communicated that fact to the patient, nor was there any record of the condition on his chart.

In all, we came to the conclusion that the care was inadequate (or worse) in more that 90 percent of the clinics we visited.

Meanwhile, there was reason to believe that fraud, waste, and abuse were accelerating and had begun to penetrate the establishment. Where once the most likely target for one of our investigations was a fringe physician – a foreign medical graduate, marginally educated, working in a marginal area – now, increasingly, frauds were found in mainstream medicine. The crooks were getting bigger. The frauds were becoming bolder, the crimes more outrageous.

A Fifth Avenue pediatrician gave an antibiotic to his neighbor's dog and charged medicaid for the service.

A psychologist indicted by the state for eight counts of theft was also found, under the guise of providing assistance, to have advised a thirteen-year-old boy to engage in both bisexual and homosexual acts. He instructed the boy how to perform both.

A hospital in Orange County maintained a full-time massage parlor for physicians, complete with erotic pictures and private rooms. The comfort station was charged to the taxpayer.

A nineteen-year-old nurse's aide in Wisconsin was charged with forcing feces into the mouth of a sixty-nine-year-old female patient who had a bowel movement at an inconvenient time. The same aide had previously held a knife to another patient's throat and threatened to kill her. In her defense, she said the woman was always asking for things and would not be quiet.

One of the physicians we interviewed in preparing for our visits had been practicing in Oregon. He returned home to New York and applied to the medicaid program only to find he had already been admitted. Somebody had borrowed his name. What bothered the doctor the most was the fact that the imposter had been pulling in $50,000 a year.

In Ohio, the chief auditor in the state's Bureau of Fiscal Affairs was indicted for accepting bribes from a nursing home operator, a well-known pediatrician plead guilty to selling Seconal and Preludin to narcotics officers, and a member of a legislative task force on the enforcement of nursing home regulations was indicted for embezzling $73,000 from patients at her home.

In North Carolina, a police chief's wife plead guilty to embezzlement from nursing home patients.

In Baton Rouge, a former state director of hospitals, along with another state official, was indicted on twenty counts of fraud.

In Spokane, a state representative was convicted of theft, embezzlement, and medicaid fraud.

A California health group was indicted for illegally siphoning more than $5 million from medicaid.

A psychologist was indicted for submitting phoney bills totalling $110,000 for service to thirty families he did not see. After further review, the state wound up suing to recover some $1.5 million from the doctor, who had been one of the leading medicaid billers in the state.

The owners of a nursing home in Wisconsin charged the government for their honeymoon in Hawaii, household improvements, and health insurance for three people not involved in the home's operation.

One of their competitors, not to be outdone, charged the government with repairs to a personal residence, for personal appliances, groceries for the administrator's family, payments for four personal cars, and for travel of a softball team they sponsored.

A third Wisconsin operator was kind enough to share the administrative costs of a tavern, two bakeries, and six beauty shops with the government. He also spent $20,000 of the state's money to support the star pitcher of his baseball team.

In Oklahoma, two brothers, one of whom served on the state's board of mental health while the other served as president of the school board, admitted they were ripping off the government.

In Hawaii, we found high-ranking state officials, including several supreme court judges, who were put on a nursing home's payroll. They were listed as janitors – well-paid janitors.

In California, we found one of the largest alcohol treatment chains in the country was recruiting its patients from the bowery and "churning" them. Skid row bums were picked up by ambulance, detoxed in California, flown to other states, and detoxed again in order to avoid screens and escape the government's payment limits.

One of them, a sixty-six-year-old man, was put on a "champagne" flight to Las Vegas after treatment in California. Another patient, a young retarded woman, was treated seven times in six different hospitals in three states in less than a year.

In the same month, a division of Revlon, Inc., was found guilty of overbilling medicaid to the tune of half a million dollars, and a millionaire pioneer of nuclear medicine plead guilty to ripping off the government for more than $50,000.

Based on these and other incidents, we had begun increasing our estimates of the amount of fraud, waste, and abuse in government health programs. We were now estimating that at least one-fourth of the money the government spent on health was either wasted or stolen.

We had come to the conclusion that fraud, waste, and abuse had permeated the program. In an analogy appropriate to the industry, the cancer had metastasized. It was spreading through the system.

Joe Ingber and his partner Shelly Styles made the point. For a while, they ran a string of clinics in New York. Styles was rotund and reticent. Ingber was smaller and forthcoming. He felt the government was cheating *him*. "Here we were asked to provide a service and, at the same time, we were being paid less that 50 percent of what we asked from a private patient," he said.

Ingber was a chiropractor. He had been recently been found guilty of stealing from the government. As a part of his plea bargain, he had agreed to cooperate with the government.

"How did it begin?"

Styles said, "We heard it was going on not only in our profession but in every one of the medical and paramedical professions."

He was middle-aged, dark, and brooding. Confession did not come easily for him.

"Doctors were writing down extra visits here and there and there was no problem with it. The worst thing that would happen is that somebody might ask you to give some of it back."

The eight medical centers Ingber and Styles controlled had grossed over $2 million in three years. The U.S. Attorney said at least half of it was stolen.

"Can you give us an example?"

"Sure," Ingber said. "One doctor billed $10,000 for ten members of one family. They called him down and said, 'Hey look. You have got to keep the families down. No more than two children a family at one time.' In a sense they were saying: It's all right to write false billing for two children, but don't make us look bad. Spread it out guys."

Probably one of the reasons Styles was less forthcoming is that he was not a doctor. He had graduated from the Chiropractic Institute of New York, but had not been able to pass the licensing exam.

Asked how he began practicing medicine, he said Dr. Ingber had asked him to join his practice during a social visit.

"He invited me to join him in his practice during a purely social visit."

"Did you also practice with Dr. Andrew Portoguese?"

"Yes."

"How did that happen?"

"I went to his office to get some records. I spoke with him and met his mother. After a while, he asked if I would like to make some extra money."

He smiled and looked at his partner.

"He asked me if I knew the neurological signs and I said, 'Yes.' Then he brought the first patient in and began doing an examination."

"What was the patient's problem?"

"The patient said he had a cold. Before I knew it, I heard Dr. Portoguese's mother say, "Don't worry. Dr. Schweiker will take care of your cold and I was thrust into the role of Dr. Schweiker."

"You posed as a medical doctor?"

"Yes. That was my first experience."

"Did you do any other examinations as Dr. Schweiker?"

"Yes, I saw the rest of the patients that evening."

"Who wrote the prescriptions?"

"Dr. Portoguese's mother wrote the prescriptions and signed Dr. Schweiker's name."

"Who was Dr. Schweiker?"

"A senile psychiatrist."

"Did you make arrangements to get some of Dr. Portoguese's patients?"

"Yes."

"How did the arrangement work?"

"We gave him a couple of dollars for each patient."

Styles mopped his brow.

"We would write up a treatment plan, begin treating them, and attempt to get their families in."

"How many visits were in your treatment plan?"

"Usually, we asked for nine to twelve for an adult. A little less for a child."

"Did this request have anything to do with their actual physical condition? Who would write the treatment plan?"

Ingber, tired of being left out, responded. "Whoever was ready would pull a treatment plan off the top and begin to write down symptoms that would be appropriate for a given person. If there wasn't a condition, we would invent one."

"We tried not to have all the treatment plans reflect the same condition," Styles added. "We tried to keep them different."

"What percentage of these treatment plans were fabricated?"

"A great percentage," Styles said.

Ingber added, "I would say more than half."

"What happened next?"

"After the treatment plan was prepared two secretaries wrote invoices indicating the dates of visits for the next few weeks, held them until the last visit date and sent them in."

"Did you actually see these patients?"

"In some cases, yes."

"Did you get a kickback from the other physicians who practiced in your clinics?"

"Yes. If they billed one hundred dollars worth of paper, they would pay us thirty dollars. If they had a 40 percent deal, they would pay us forty dollars out of every one hundred."

"What makes the difference between a 30 percent and a 40 percent deal?"

"Supply and demand. If we needed somebody badly, we might make a better deal with him. By and large, an internist or pediatrician or others that the patients wanted the most would get the best deal."

"How about Dr. Yood?"

We had been told Dr. Yood was mentally confused.

"He was on salary. We paid him $200 a week."

"Why was he there?"

"By and large he was there so we could use him."

"What percentage of his bills were false?"

"Around 90 percent."

Ingber admitted they drove Yood from clinic to clinic just so he could sign blank invoices indicating he had seen patients in each clinic.

"Do doctors trade patients?"

"It was very common for one doctor to finish billing a patient and another doctor to start billing the same patient."

"What's this practice called?"

"Ping-ponging."

"Is it widespread?"

"Every clinic I know about is doing it," Styles said.

"Everybody's bragging about it, too," Ingber added.

"It was like finding a wallet. If you find a wallet on the street with $100 bills in it, what are you going to do, turn your back and ignore it?"

Ingber offered some advice.

"If you want to set up a system that is going to be corrupt, start out by underpaying the practitioner. At the same time, make it very easy for them to cheat, don't put in any safeguards, and then turn you back on the whole system and walk away from it."

He had a point.

"What you are trying to do is put your finger in the dike. The whole system is impossible."

We knew he was right.

We were past the point where some limited action would be effective. We needed a coordinated comprehensive strike, some mechanism that would focus the government's policing efforts. We had settled on creation of an inspector general – a "supercop" who would be given responsibility for cleaning up the mess in medicare and medicaid.

We knew, too, that if we were to have any chance of success, we had to move fast. But speed is not one of Congress' strong points. At that time, members introduced about 1,000 pieces of legislation a year. Less than one hundred were enacted and most of them were routine measures (funding bills), or had been kicking around Congress in variations for years.

As an investigative committee, our road was even longer and the obstacles greater because any measure we developed would have to be referred to other committees for consideration and action. No matter how worthy the measure, politics, practice, and tradition demanded the legislative committees give precedence to their own agendas.

The only effective antidote we had found to this bureaucratic inertia was the judicious use of the natural phenomena – heat and light. We found if we applied enough light to the subject, the heat of public opinion would force action. In a word, we were embarrassing the committees into doing their jobs.

Congressional inertia is caused by the first law of politics, which is to avoid organized opposition whenever possible. We were balancing the peril a member faces when he or she votes for a measure that will offend some group with an effective lobby, with the hazard of offending a larger constituency if they do not.

It is no accident, therefore, that we came to measure the success of our activities by exposure – how many cameras were at the hearing, how many page-one stories, how many above the fold, how many follow-up calls, how many features and related stories, and how much air time our stories received.

It was also no accident that the one question we were most frequently asked in our pre-hearing briefings was, "How many cameras?"

Rule of thumb: You can count on at least one member present for every camera at the hearing. In an age when most hearings drew two or three members, we averaged ten to twenty. To this date, my brother and I hold both the House and Senate records for number of cameras present at staff-generated events.

Over the years, we had achieved a fair degree of success as our efforts gained more and more prominence. We had established a track record of front page stories that drew national attention. Our investigations routinely made the evening news and were the subject of features in news magazines of the three networks.

We knew the kind of activity we were engaged in would draw national attention, but given the stakes we decided to up the ante. We asked the chairman if he would give us a day of his time. To be reasonably safe, we asked Joe Hynes for backup.

Joe Hynes is a man of complete integrity. Whenever the state of New York is in trouble and needs someone to clean up a particularly sticky mess, they call for

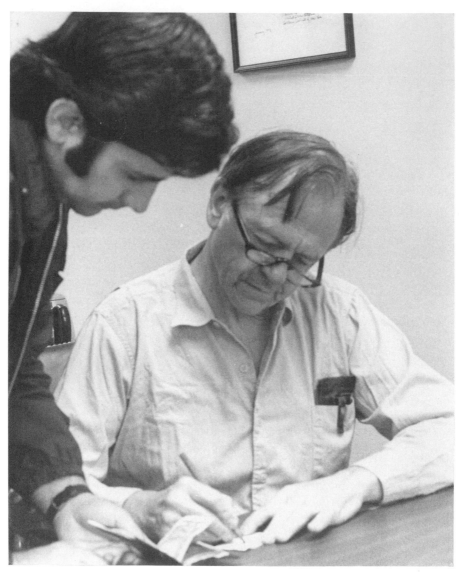

photo by Val Halamandaris
Senator Moss signing his medicaid card.

Joe. It's one of the few consistent signs of intelligence in New York government.

At the time, in the wake of the Bergman incident, Hynes was Deputy Attorney General for Medicaid Fraud Control. We asked him for backup while Senator Moss was on the street and in harm's way. We also asked for the wireless.

Hynes could scarcely contain his delight when our party arrived in his office. "You'll have to pardon me, Senator," he said. "I'm just a poor Irishman. I never thought I'd see a U.S. Senator dressed like this."

In addition to his khakis and the denim jacket he wore, Moss had on a pair of sneakers and an old baseball hat. The medicaid card he had just signed was in his back pocket along with a phoney social security card I had just picked up on the street. Both read "F. Edward Moss."

The ends of a small brown bag protruded from the pocket of his jacket. It contained a half pint of Boone's Farm Grape, obtained to complete his disguise. The bottle had been purchased at a liquor store on Chamber Street where the margin between clients and clerks is nearly indistinguishable.

We'd been coming into this shop for months. Each time, I asked for a receipt to satisfy the committee's somewhat anal chief clerk. Each time, the proprietor humored me by writing a receipt to the U.S. Senate for 90 cents without showing any reaction. This time his eyes grew wide as our entourage descended on his store.

"I know you can't talk now," he said, surveying the odd collection of suits, street clothes, cameras, and recorders. "But some day will you come by just long enough to tell me what's going on?"

I told him he would know in a few days.

As Moss came out of the clinic in East Harlem, an assortment of cameras recorded the event. We filmed his walk to the pharmacy where he filled the half dozen prescriptions he had been given and taped his running commentary.

"Looks like I have a sore throat. I may have meningitis. Dr. Carey will be surprised."

Dr. Carey, the Physician of the Capitol, had certified Moss' good health two days earlier.

"At the very least, I should cut back on my drinking."

Moss, a Mormon, drank very little.

"It's absolutely outrageous. Allergy tests, chest x-rays, urine tests, and four physicians in less than thirty minutes."

Most of that had occurred while he waited to see the first doctor.

"You are right, guys, volume is the key. No wonder they're called 'medicaid mills.'"

A week later, to a packed house in the historic Senate Caucus Room, Moss expressed his outrage. "Medicaid isn't medicine. It's business. Curing patients is good medicine, but bad business."

"If you are not sick, you won't be told you're not sick. If you are sick, the odds are you won't be helped."

The story played on the front page of every newspaper in the country. Clips of our home movies were used by all three networks and the Senate seemed stunned by the graphic detail of our findings.

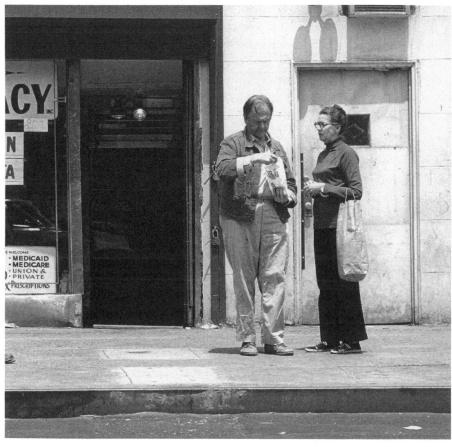

photo by Val Halamandaris
Senator Moss leaving a welfare clinic.

David Matthews responded for the administration. "Moss is grandstanding," he said and dismissed the matter.

Jimmy Carter, then in the middle of his campaign for the presidency, picked up the gauntlet. He accused the Nixon and Ford administrations of ignoring documented charges of fraud, waste, and corruption in medicare and medicaid for years. Carter cited our findings as "a terrible example of federal bureaucratic indifference."

Chapter Four
Crime Without Punishment
———❦———

By every account, Richard Kones was a brilliant physician. He was also a brilliant crook.

In the fall of 1982, Kones appeared before a rare joint session of two Senate committees. "From 1977 until the fall of 1980, Dr. Kones, you submitted over $1.5 million in false claims for services you never rendered," Senator Dole said. "Is that correct, Doctor?"

"Yes."

Kones had also bilked the Labor Department's Workman's Compensation Program, and several private insurance companies during the same period.

"Apparently, you did this by simply changing the service dates and sending in the identical bill for payment?"

"Yes sir."

"Did you also defraud social security?" Senator Heinz asked.

"Yes."

In May of 1979, Kones had admitted himself to a hospital complaining of chest pains. He brought with him doctored blood tests and an EKG indicating heart problems. Two days later, he checked out of the hospital and started taking tennis lessons.

"On June 25, on the basis of a cardiologist's analysis of the phoney tests, you applied for social security disability."

"Yes sir."

Kones looked increasingly uncomfortable. He had deep-set dark eyes that did not appear to enjoy the light of a dozen cameras.

"How much did you receive?"

"A thousand a month for nineteen months."

"Did you also file a disability claim with your personal insurance carrier?"

"Yes."

"How much did you receive?"

"About a quarter of a million."

"In 1974 you were indicted and convicted in New York. What were the charges?"

"Medicare fraud."

"What was your sentence?"

"Five years' probation."

"When did you resume fraudulent activities?"

"The bulk of my fraudulent activities did not occur until 1978."

"I find it absolutely incredible that you were convicted in 1974 and committed the bulk of these offenses while you were still on probation," Senator Heinz said. "You were not only allowed to continue practicing, but it took them six years to find out what you were doing."

Kones was consulting editor to three medical journals. He had authored four books, had a legitimate income in excess of $100,000, and was listed in *Who's Who in North America.*

He had begun his criminal activities within two years of graduation from medical school. By all evidence those activities had continued, essentially without change, for more than ten years.

In the wake of our investigation of medicaid mills, Congress had enacted sweeping reforms. As we had hoped one bill established an Office of the Inspector General for the Department of Health, Education and Welfare – the first Inspector General's Office for any federal department, and the model for the thirteen others that would subsequently be created.

A second provision authorized the creation of state medicaid fraud units, which would receive funding from the federal government. The efforts of the state fraud units were to be facilitated and coordinated by the Office of the Inspector General.

In addition, the administration of medicare and medicaid was to be unified in a new department, the Health Care Financing Administration. Among other things, it was thought the unification of administrative responsibility would centralize all of the department's fraud-fighting capacity in one office, providing the inspector general (IG) with enough resources to properly attack systemic abuse.

In arguing for the creation of the office, Senator Moss had cited the statistics: In 1976, there were a total of 123 people in medicare's program integrity unit. These people were spread out in ten regional offices, with a headquarters in Baltimore. If you did the math, it worked out to about one man to validate every $115.5 million being spent by the program.

There were additionally ten trained investigators who focused on the $15 billion federal share of medicaid. One of them called us in early 1976. He made a strange request. He wanted to talk – but not in the office. He asked if we could meet him somewhere private.

In confidence, he spoke of the millions in fraud and potential fraud cases backlogged at the department. He said he wanted a "friend on the Hill." He said he was frustrated by the system.

Inadvertently, he said, the security unit of his office had offended a powerful Senate staffer. The department had investigated what appeared to be a junket taken by an employee at public expense. The allegation was that the employee had collected on both ends, taking money from her hosts while charging the government for her expenses at the same time.

The employee in question was the staffer's wife. The committee he worked for controlled appropriations. In retaliation, or perhaps with some broader motive, he

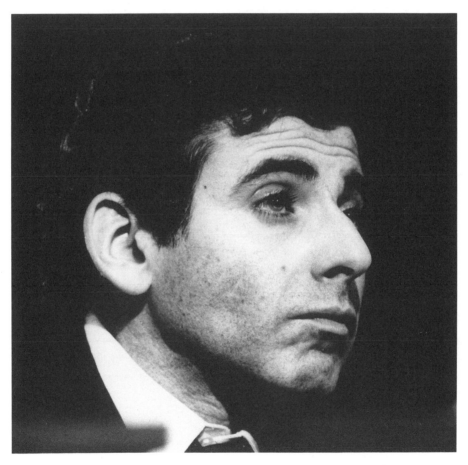

photo by Bill Halamandaris
"The system is extremely easy to evade." –Dr. Richard Kones

had slashed the security branch's budget and, in an effort to control security, had curtailed investigations as well.

"Because of the limitations in manpower," Moss said in a floor statement, "only 400 of the 10,000 cases filed against physicians through the years have been investigated and referred to the Justice Department for prosecution.

"If the chances that a case will be developed are slim the odds of prosecution are slimmer still, and the chances of being found guilty are incalculable. Less than 1.5 percent of all accused physicians in fraud cases have been found guilty.

"The chances of a physician going to jail are barely measurable. Only fifteen doctors have done jail time related to medicare and medicaid fraud since the beginning of the program ten years ago. The chances of a doctor having his license revoked or being terminated from participation in those programs are non-existent. Only two physicians have lost their licenses and none have been terminated from either medicare or medicaid in the history of those programs."

The worst thing that had happened to the worst offenders was that they were asked to pay back some of the money they had stolen. It seemed a strange sort of punishment – a government-subsidized, interest-free loan.

One of those convicted was a doctor in New Jersey who was charging medicare for the removal of cancerous lesions. Investigators found he had removed harmless warts in twenty-one of twenty-three cases. He plead guilty to thirteen felony counts. He was fined $1,000, placed on probation for two years, and forced to endure a stern lecture.

"It's astonishing that a man of your standing in the community, whose income is many times that of the average citizen, should stoop to this theft from the United States government," the judge said. "It's unbelievable. I will not sentence you to prison although I thought about it."

A California podiatrist billed for performing serious surgery on half a dozen patients – surgery that included the removal of several bones that could not have grown back. Investigators found he had instead been clipping the patients' toenails. He plead guilty and was released because the court said there was no evidence he was continuing to commit these crimes.

A Florida physician billed for office visits while he was vacationing in Europe. He received a suspended sentence. So did the chiropractor who was convicted of billing medicaid for manipulating the spines of people who were dead or in prison.

George Wilson, then Assistant U.S. Attorney for the Southern District of New York, called with great excitement one morning. He had made a breakthrough, he said. One of his docs was going to do "hard time."

I asked how long.

"Two months of weekends."

In order to obtain the conviction, Wilson had reconstructed the physician's payment records by hand. He had commandeered free labor, pressing into service half a dozen conscientious objectors to sort through the thousands of invoices chaotically stored in the government's warehouse.

It seemed like the juice hardly justified the squeeze, and I said so.

"Listen," he replied. "You should know by now you just don't put a doctor in jail unless he kills somebody and then only if he or she used a gun."

In the post-Bergman era, Joe Hynes successfully prosecuted ninety-four health care crooks. Only one received a sentence longer than four years. In total, they had stolen more than $50 million from the public. Hynes recovered $8 million of that total.

Medical fraud had become so endemic, the process was being taught. We taped one physician who was running his own "school for scoundrels."

"If they ask you, all you tell them is 'We're interested in good medicine'," he said. "That's all you have to say. What are they going to do? I don't know what you did in your practice. You don't know what I did in mine. The nurse, is she going to argue with you? Besides, she won't even be in the room when you see the patient. So it comes down to the patient. He's going to say what? At worst, it comes down to his word against yours. If they ask you, 'Did you ever put down for a patient you didn't see?' you say, 'I don't recall.' If they ask you, 'Would you do that?' you say, 'No, that's dishonest. I wouldn't even think about it.' 'Did you do these procedures?' 'Yes, but that's not my handwriting. The girl did the work. I should read it more carefully.' There is no way to prove a thing. Even if they show you the worst piece of paper you ever wrote, there's no way to prove a thing."

That was the kind of thing the Inspector General's Office was supposed to stop – with the broad power of the new law, the mandate that administration of medicare and medicaid should be improved by centralizing responsibility, and the pre-election commitment of the Carter administration. We had hoped for more. Instead, the problems continued.

The first prosecution in the state of Oklahoma for medicaid fraud – some twelve years after the program was enacted – resulted in an order to repay a fraction of the amount the owners of a nursing home were proven to have stolen. A thirty-five-year-old physician in Tennessee was accused of 300 counts of medicare and medicaid fraud. The prosecutors charged the physician had engaged in a "constant, deliberate, repeated pattern of fraud" resulting in the theft of more than $1 million from the government. He was convicted on eighty-two counts and sentenced to ten months.

A psychiatrist in Wisconsin got off even lighter. He was released on probation with the explanation that "fear of maximal punishment might have the effect of deterring psychiatrists from accepting medicaid patients."

In North Carolina, a dentist who had received the second highest amount of medicaid money in the state the year before was indicted on thirty-one felony counts. Under the new law, he could have received a maximum sentence of ten years for each count. He was given a five-year suspended sentence and ordered to spend sixteen hours in community service.

The first doctor convicted in Hawaii spent his entire thirty-day jail sentence in a state hospital after his psychiatrist convinced the court the physician had developed a heart problem and "an irrational fear of jail."

A pharmacist in Ohio admitted he had stolen $83,000 from government programs. He was sentenced to ninety days in jail and fined $2,500.

The owner of a Milwaukee nursing home was charged with fifty-eight felony counts, including one charge of homicide by negligence. He had previously been convicted on kickback charges and was reputed to operate a facility that "would shock the human conscience." He, too, received a ninety-day sentence and a fine. The fine was the amount the government could *prove* he had stolen.

A few months later, a Maryland pediatrician received a similar sentence. He was given an option of paying a $10,000 fine or giving 200 hours of free work to the county.

The largest fraud detected in the history of the Maryland program resulted in an order to pay back $112,314 and complete 300 hours of community service. The *Evening Sun* supported the sentence on the theory that incarcerating the physician would "deprive society in general and his patients in particular of professional services in short supply."

A Utah district judge provided the best rationale for not sending a physician to jail. Aggravated by the psychiatrist's lack of forthrightness, the judge said he was "afraid to sentence the doctor to jail out of fear he might corrupt the criminals."

Joe Hynes provided the best evidence of the lack of progress. Four years after the Inspector General's Office had been created, Hynes repeated our medicaid investigation, sending undercover agents into medicaid clinics and pharmacies throughout New York City. In less than three months, investigators identified $3 million in fraud and indicted thirty-nine people.

About the same time, the FBI got into the act. Drawn by the publicity and the importance Congress had placed on cleaning up health programs, the Bureau began an undercover operation that "would have a high probability of success and would be the most effective way to not only determine the depth of the problem but, with minimal use of manpower, would enable the investigators to obtain direct evidence of the crimes being committed."

In other words, they did what we had done years before. FBI agents posed as businessmen interested in the health care industry. "It was immediately apparent," their spokesman said, "that kickbacks, rebates, and fraud were a way of life."

In the first three months of the operation, the FBI opened twenty-two cases. They received kickbacks from hospitals, nursing homes, clinics, doctors, and clinical laboratories. They came to the conclusion that "no phase of the medicare or medicaid programs was free from fraud."

Bud Mullens, speaking for the Bureau, testified that the abuses identified by Senate staffers before the creation of the Inspector General's Office were still occurring and had "apparently become more widespread."

"We learned many things from the investigation," Mullen said, "the most evident of which is that corruption has permeated virtually every area of medicare and medicaid. The people committing these frauds have absolutely no fear of being caught. The people who commit these frauds are aware of their illegal activity; however, they have decided to take the risk because they believe that if they are caught, the worst thing that will happen to them is that they will have to repay the money they obtained fraudulently."

Privately, Mullen, then Assistant Director of the FBI's Criminal Investigation Unit, told us he had never seen anything like it in his twenty years with the Bureau. "The fraud was obvious, rampant, and outlandish."

In one instance, he said a doctor was paid $2 million in a two-year period for medicare and medicaid activities. He was found to have been performing abortions on women who were not pregnant.

"This doctor billed for an abortion he performed on a woman who had previously had a hysterectomy. He said he performed another on a woman who previously had a tubal ligation. In forty-eight separate instances, this doctor had billed for performing two abortions within one month on the same patients."

"While conducting this investigation," he said, "it was discovered that two doctors were racing to determine who could perform the most abortions in a day. They kept track by putting check marks on their surgical gowns, which were not changed between abortions.

"In another instance we found a case where a kickback of $100,000 was given to a doctor for $140,000 worth of supplies ordered by a hospital."

Ironically, the operation was closed down, Mullen testified, because it was too successful. "We could have gone further but we had to cease our operations because we were having difficulty preparing the cases for court. It got to the point where we were in over our heads."

Before they began the undercover operation, the Bureau had 230 medicare and medicaid fraud cases pending nationally. Within a few months, their case load had tripled to 684 cases.

"In Los Angeles (where the FBI sting had taken place), we found we burdened the U.S. Attorney's Office with 160 cases. They said they could handle maybe four a month."

Expenditures for health in the years since the creation of the Inspector General's Office had increased by more than 65 percent. The IG's best guess was that fraud, waste, and abuse had increased twice as fast during the same period. Where did we go wrong?

The Inspector General's Office had been modeled on Joe Hynes' operation in New York. After the legislation passed the Senate, Secretary Mathews and his people descended on the House. They ware aided by the Department of Justice and the American Medical Association. The Department of Justice expressed concern about the creation of a new police force and assured the House they could do the job. The AMA lobbied against the bill on principle, saying it wasn't needed and that the problem was overstated.

As a result, the Democratic House acceded to the requests of the Republican administration. Two key provisions were deleted from the Senate bill. The House agreed the IG should be a political appointee under the supervision of the secretary of the department he or she was to inspect. They also agreed to eliminate the provision that would have empowered the inspector general to go directly to court with its cases when the Justice Department declined prosecution.

The inspector general was boxed in. Without control of his or her own budget and resources, without independent authority and access to the courts, there was little the IG could do. We would have been better off creating a temporary ad hoc committee to study the problem. At least then we would have been assured continuity. Everyone knows the closest thing to immortality on earth is a temporary congressional committee.

About the time we were ready to despair, the problem was solved. With one stroke, Patricia Harris, then Secretary of Health, Education and Welfare eliminated fraud, waste, and abuse. The secretary decreed the terms "fraud, waste, and abuse" would be banned from the department's dictionary, sweeping the problem out of her domain and under the rug. The secretary said she preferred the more antiseptic terms "program misuse" and "mismanagement."

Ronald Reagan was among those who were not impressed. Reagan made efficiency in government a major focus of his campaign. He decried the waste in public programs and singled out the Department of Health, Education and Welfare for special attention. Reagan cited our estimates of loss to the program and the cost to the taxpayer and pledged a Reagan administration would do better.

He sounded a lot like Carter had four years earlier.

Despite Reagan's pledge and his commitment to make government more efficient, our review indicated the Inspector General's Office was operating at a disquieting level of inactivity. Rather than complete the consolidation of anti-fraud activities and dedicate the resources necessary to do the job, the administration began cutting back across the board. There were still forty-three other agencies within the department with significant responsibility for preventing and prosecuting fraud, waste, and abuse.

As a result, in 1981 the State of New York had as many criminal investigators as the inspector general had for the entire nation. The IG had referred all of forty-one cases for prosecution. In the same year, the FBI had developed several hundred cases in a few months. Only five of the IG's cases had resulted in convictions.

The inspector general's audit capacity was similarly limited. The department had a backlog of $70 million in outstanding audits even though they averaged a five dollar return for every dollar spent auditing. By comparison, New York's recovery averaged $2,500.

The state fraud units, charged with primary responsibility for policing medicaid under the IG's supervision, were equally ineffective. Eighteen states had not reported a conviction. Seven others reported a single conviction.

While we observed this trend with mounting frustration, we were faced with a startling statistic. In 1980, Blue Cross (one of medicare's intermediaries) was reporting an audit recovery ratio of 7.6 to 1 – seven plus dollars recovered for every dollar spent. Two years later, they were reporting a recovery rate of twenty-six to one. In some parts of the country, notably California and New York, the ratio was even higher, approaching fifty dollars recovered for every audit dollar spent.

The best estimate in 1965 was that by the year 1990 medicare costs would reach $9 billion. Actual expenses in 1990 approached ten times that projection. Some of that excess was due to inflation. But a lot of it was the result of fraud and abuse. Even more was wasted in money that, while not stolen, was needlessly spent.

No wonder the Health, Education and Welfare investigator who wanted a "friend on the Hill" was shocked. "We all had high hopes," he said, "but nothing's changed in the way they've handled fraud and abuse. There's a new department, an Inspector General's Office, but it's just there. Nothing has changed. They are ignoring the law."

Richard Kones, M.D. reinforced the point. "The forms I sent in were absolutely outrageous," he said

"What do you mean?" Senator Heinz asked.

"I made a list of sixteen flags on the forms, sixteen features that should have alerted authorities to what I was doing. The system is that vulnerable."

"That's absolutely remarkable," Heinz said with disgust. "Sixteen different flags. Somebody convicted in 1974, and it still took six years to find it."

"Unfortunately, the system is extremely easy to evade."

"Did anybody representing any agency of the government ever inquire of you in any way as to whether or not you had a prior criminal record?" Senator Mitchell asked.

"No sir."

"How much time did you do for the crimes for which you were sentenced in 1974?" the former federal judge continued.

"Thirty days."

"You stole hundreds of thousands of dollars and ended up with a thirty-day sentence. That strikes me as incredible. I've sentenced men to jail for two to three to five years for stealing less than $1,000."

"Were any of them doctors?" Kones asked and seemed shaken by the thought.

Watching his reaction, I remembered the day we met. He had been in the Tombs for the night. While he waited for the marshals, two other inmates found reason to quarrel. Apparently the argument had to do with ear distribution because at its conclusion one inmate had three and the other only one. The victor carried the extra ear in his teeth until he was restrained. Kones had been pressed into to service to reattach the separated ear.

"That's not supposed to make any difference, " Mitchell said. "We are supposed to have a system in which all people are treated equally before the law. It's not just the poor and minorities who are supposed to spend time in jail."

Richard Kusserow was called on to respond. Kusserow had been plucked from the ranks of the FBI by President Reagan to head the Inspector General's Office. We thought we were doing him a favor by giving him an excuse to reorganize the office, and some ammunition to use in gathering additional resources.

For some reason, Kusserow didn't agree. The night before he appeared, I had given his liaison a copy of our report. The aide, fearful of his boss' reaction, had not shared it with him until just before the hearing. Kusserow thanked me for it in private, commenting it was his birthday and saying that I had given him a birthday present he would long remember.

The two congressional committees most concerned about cleaning up medicare and medicaid were primed and ready, but Kusserow couldn't pull the trigger. A career FBI man, he could not divorce himself from the office he had inherited. A loyalist, he could not break ranks with the administration by asking for additional resources, though privately he would acknowledge the necessity.

The day before the joint hearing, the administration called a preemptive press conference to show how well the fifteen inspector generals were doing. The president announced these watchdogs had saved the taxpayers $2 billion in the

the previous year. Proudly, the president concluded his inspector generals were "meaner than a junk yard dog."

If it was meant to blunt the impact of our investigation, it had the opposite effect, setting Kusserow up. After examining the record, Senator David Pryor, a gentle man, couldn't help noting that the IG looked less like a junk yard dog than a "pet kitten."

Pryor has a long history of concern for the elderly. Along with Senator Heinz, he was instrumental as a congressman in the formation of the House Aging Committee. When they encountered opposition, they set up a trailer in the parking lot, calling it the House Special Committee on Aging and operating on an ad hoc basis until the leadership was embarrassed into formalizing the activity.

At one point early on, Pryor had spent a few weeks working in a nursing home to see firsthand what it was like. He knew about the historical abuses of the program. He spoke out of frustration many shared.

"What has been evidenced here today," he said, "is that you invite fraud and abuse by a laxity of enforcement, a laxity of interest and oversight. You invite it. When you have that kind of profit – millions of dollars – with little risk of being detected, then you are inviting abuse."

"There is a more fundamental problem," Kusserow responded. "We had an underlying assumption that the people in the helping professions could be relied upon to follow the Hippocratic (or other similar ethical) oath. Were that a valid premise, we wouldn't have to develop the kind of controls you would in other sectors. We have found that was not a valid assumption."

Chapter Five
Everybody's a Wise Guy
——❦——

"I was in medicaid from the beginning," the doctor said.

We were in his Continental, driving through the Bronx.

"I was one of the pioneers. People thought I was crazy."

He was carrying a pearl-handled revolver in a shoulder holster. I was carrying a recorder supplied by the U.S. Attorney.

One of us is crazy, I thought. I had seen the revolver. I hoped he couldn't see the recorder.

"Up until medicaid, I never made $100,000. In my first year, I made over $200,000. Then we had a fire and the whole place burned down.

I sat on the passenger side of the front seat. His German Shepherd sat on the floor between my feet. His head was inches from my crotch.

"I hope you were covered."

"Oh, yeah."

He wore a two-toned, iridescent, three-piece suit. His maroon shoes were made of patent leather.

A few days earlier, I had answered an advertisement in the *New York Times*. "I'm Tom Clancey with Total Health Care," I said. "I'm interested in buying your clinic."

The receptionist asked me to hold. In a moment a male responded.

"Dr. Port. Who is this?" He had a flat nasal voice.

I repeated the fictitious name I had selected for this stunt, wondering again why I always pick on the Irish.

"Who'd you say you're with?"

"I'm the east coast representative of Total Health Care."

"Where are you from?"

"Chicago. Are you the one selling the clinic?"

"Yeah."

"I'd like to come out and talk to you."

He agreed and we made an appointment for the following afternoon.

That afternoon I found a cut-rate printer and had business cards made up listing Total Health Care Industries, Inc., a Chicago address, my fictitious name, and the number of the telephone the General Service Administration had wired into my room at the Algonquin.

I went through our target file and pulled his records. He had in fact made over $200,000 each year since the beginning of the program. He had been the subject of grand jury investigation in 1972 and had been reviewed frequently by the city health department. His file was three inches thick.

Despite a number of complaints and investigations, he had never been suspended or disciplined by the program. He had not been indicted by the grand jury in 1972. Nor did he have a record of any subsequent prosecution.

The records did indicate that, from time to time, he could be hard to find. The day-to-day operation of the facility was handled by an administrator. It was believed he had other medical operations in the south, but this fact had not been confirmed.

I could have confirmed it if they had asked me.

I got George Wilson, the Assistant U.S. Attorney on the phone, told him what was going on, and asked if I could borrow a recorder. He agreed, with the stipulation that he had the right to field any criminal cases that came out of our inquiry.

In the morning when I arrived at Manhattan South, Wilson was in court. He had left a note telling me to ask for Carl Bogan. I passed the note to the receptionist and waited a few minutes while she rang inside.

A few moments later a tall, bald, ageless man came forward from the inner sanctum.

"Carl Bogan." He stuck out a big, meaty hand.

"Do you want a KEL or the Nagra?"

Bogan had worked as a cop for some thirty years in New York. He had worked all the rackets, first for the city, then for the D.A., and now for the U.S. Attorney. Over his desk was a picture of Telly Savalas. The picture was autographed, "To Kojak from Kojak."

He asked where I was going, what the circumstances would be, and how long I would be out. When I explained we were trying to mousetrap one of the wise guys, he smiled a big, beautiful smile.

"Sounds like you'd better take the Nagra. It's a bit bulkier, but you're big enough to carry it and it has twice the life."

He opened a desk drawer and pulled out what looked to be a pocket warmer sewn into a canvas belt.

"You can either wear it under your arm, sling it, or wrap it around your waist."

He demonstrated.

"I generally clip it inside the belt of my pants. Put the recorder in the small of your back. I run the cord down my trouser leg."

He held up about three feet of cord attached to a small mushroom-shaped microphone.

"Cut a hole in the bottom of one pocket and feed the control right up through. There's just one thing. Once you start it, push this tape over and seal it. Don't try to start it and stop it to save tape."

He smiled.

"For one thing, you can't keep your hand in your pocket forever – even in this town. But more important, if the tape cuts in and out, it's dead. We'll never be able to use it in court. Got it?"

I said I did.

"You want a backup or one of our agents to carry the wire?"

"No."

"Personal?"

I nodded.

"What time is your appointment?"

"Three."

"Give me a call later and let me know how it went."

Later, outside the Bronx clinic, I thumbed the machine on and went in. After experimenting in the hotel, I had taped the recorder to the back of my right calf.

We were in the part of town that used to be known as "Fort Apache." The police station steps still bore the stains of the blood spilled there a couple of years earlier when the place was under siege. Now it is known as the "Little House on the Prairie." The station is the only thing standing for miles. Four out of every five buildings on any given block in that area have been burned and gutted.

Only a few brick buildings stood intact and half of these seemed to be welfare clinics like the one I entered. Inside was dark, dusty, and depressing. A number of young, apparently healthy young men milled around nervously waiting to be called.

At first Port seemed suspicious. He took me on a quick tour of the facility after examining my card explaining, "I'm really rushed right now. I have an appointment downtown."

I asked him about the operation.

"The way I run this place, my administrator goes around and makes sure that patients see practically everybody and everybody keeps constantly busy."

"What do you have to pay the docs?"

"They pay me. I get $1,000 a month from the dentist and the pharmacist and $1,500 from the podiatrist and the chiropractor. The internist pays $2,000 a month."

"That's it."

"No. We split everything they bill sixty-forty."

"Who gets sixty?"

"You do."

"Do they have a piece of management?"

He shook his head in disgust.

"No. They're puppets. They're just here. They're workers and you're the boss. They're all on oral agreements. If I don't like them, they are out."

He made me wonder how I could have asked such a dumb question. I tried another.

"What does it cost to run this place?"

"It costs $1,150 a month plus utilities."

"What can we expect to make?"

"Half a million minimum."

"Minimum? "

"Minimum. This is medicaid-land. It's Fort Apache. Anything goes. And nobody ever bothers me."

"Sounds like a good business."

"It is. I guarantee you it's a better return on your money than Wall Street. I'll show you my books and everything, if you are really interested."

"I'd like that," I said with sincerity.

Dr. Port looked at his watch.

"Look, you've got me over a barrel. I've got another deal. Let's get together later. I'll check you out and then we can talk, okay?"

I made a mental note to shore up our flimsy cover and took a chance. I told him I had arrived by cab and asked if I could hitch a ride downtown. "Maybe we can talk some along the way."

"Great," he said with genuine enthusiasm. "That's the best idea yet. Take a ride with me."

The further we got from the clinic the more relaxed he seemed to become.

"This is the wild west out here. Everything else burns down, but our office will never burn down. You can make a nice buck in insurance though if you want to."

The recorder was beginning to cut off the circulation to my leg. I shifted positions and the dog came to attention.

"If business is so good, why do you want to get out?"

"I'm not getting out. I'm just selling this place. I have pieces of several others here in New York. I socked it away and did some good things from there. I went to Miami. I've done very well."

"Do the other clinics operate the same way?"

"Right. But in Miami it's all medicare. There's no dental. It's radiology, you know, very heavy EKGs. Everybody's into internal medicine, cardiology."

"Are there any other differences?"

"Miami is harder because you've got Americans, Jews. In New York, you've got mostly Puerto Ricans. It's a hell of a lot easier working with Puerto Ricans than Jews. Especially, old Jews – they can be very tough."

"What's the volume?"

"Half a million. If you're interested, we can work out a package deal."

I said we were interested.

"You may also want to get into the union business."

"We do some of that in Chicago. Who do you talk to out here?"

"The president of the local is Paul Peters. You give him a few bucks and he puts you on a panel."

I knew Peters. A few months back, he had wandered in the unmarked door of our Senate office.

"I hear you're looking into health frauds," he had said. "This is the guy you should go after."

He handed me a professionally prepared binder complete with tabs and an index. The binder contained a series of affidavits fingering one of his competitors, who he said was giving the labor movement a bad name.

I was so impressed with the public spirit of the small genial man, I didn't bother asking how he'd found us or why he bypassed the receptionist.

I did make a few calls and quickly found myself talking to Father Philip Carey,

Director of the Xavier Institute of Industrial Relations. Carey, I was told, had played a leading role in cleaning up the waterfront in the fifties. Some said he was the model for the priest in the movie "On the Waterfront."

"Oh, yes," he said. "I know who you mean. The boys call him Ice Pick Peters. He was Joe Current's bodyguard until Joe was killed. Some people said Peters had a hand in that."

"How did Current die?"

"Somebody put a couple of holes in his body about the size of an ice pick."

"Do you think Peters did it?"

"Whether he did or not, he wound up running the union."

"How did he get into health?"

"After a lot of trouble, the maritime people bought him out. I'm told they paid him $300,000 to leave. Apparently, he used that money to buy into the health professionals union."

"Has he gone straight?"

The priest laughed.

"What's his game, then?"

"He is said to be running a version of the protection racket. If you want to practice medicine on his turf, you've got to be a member."

The priest concluded with a note of caution. "Be careful," he said. "You're dealing with an evil man."

"How much is Peters going to want?" I asked the good doctor.

"You've got to cut your own deal. For all I know, you've got a recorder on you."

I laughed and fought the impulse to check for protrusions.

"I take it he's not going to dent the bankroll."

"Not if your bankroll is as big as you say it is."

"Anything else I should know?"

"Yes, but I've got to be careful. I was approached by a guy like you about three years ago. I had a very nice deal for him. Unfortunately, at the time there was a big war going on between Columbo and Gallo and the guy disappeared off the face of the earth."

He paused and looked directly at me.

"It's too bad. He was a beautiful guy."

We pulled into a parking garage across the street from the New York Hilton.

"Anything goes. Anything you want to do you can do. It's an unlimited situation."

"Sounds like a blank check."

"It is. A blank check for as much money as you want to make."

"Would you be willing to help me sell this to my directors?"

"If you're really interested. But I've got to know who you are first. I'm going to make a couple of calls."

We left the garage with the parking attendant eyeing the dog and trying to summon up enough courage to move the car.

"Let's talk next week. If you are on the level, we'll sit down and make a deal. I'll make you an offer you can't refuse."

I wasn't sure if he was trying to be funny. I called Bogan from a phone booth and told him what we had. He couldn't have been happier if his kid had parked one over the bleachers.

"You're beautiful. Bring the tape by in the morning and we'll get on it."

I walked the rest of the way back to the Algonquin, mulling it over. By the time I arrived, I was limping. My leg had cramped so badly, I had to cut the recorder free.

There are those, including some members of our committee, who prefer to believe that the government's health programs have somehow escaped the interest of organized crime. These same people tend to believe that professional wrestling is on the level.

In fact, allegations of mob influence are constant. Besides Gallo and Columbo, we had tied a number of the bosses to health rackets. Joe Bonanno, Sr., head of the Bonanno family was tied to health benefits plans in Arizona. Salvatore (Bill) Bonanno had been indicted for bilking the elderly in home remodeling frauds, and Jimmy (the Weasel) Fratianno had tied the Dragna family from Detroit to a series of health plans financed through the Teamsters.

These connections to the so-called Mafia were the least of our problems. There are only a few thousand (maybe 5,000) full-fledged members of the Mafia. Despite the mystique and the media hype, they are a small part of the nation's underworld. There are as many gangs in the underworld as there are consulting firms in Washington.

Somewhere along the line in every investigation we learned to expect a link to the mob. Almost as inevitably, sometime after that someone would try to pull a political lever and turn us off.

In June of 1973, the Select Committee on Crime chaired by Congressman Claude Pepper turned over an interesting tidbit in the process of investigating organized crime influence on horse racing.

Carlos Marcello, long identified as the head of syndicate operations in New Orleans, was asked what he was doing in New York at the restaurant, La Stella, in Queens in 1966.

"I went on a business trip."

"What was the nature of your business?"

"To try to get a loan on a nursing home."

With Marcello at the time were the mafia bosses Carlo Gambino, Santo Trafficante, and eleven other notorious racketeers.

Other mafia ties to nursing homes included the Bergman case in New York and the related ties of Meyer Lansky's bag man, John Pullman, to the ownership of three nursing homes in Buffalo. One of the Buffalo nursing homes was found to have stolen half a million dollars from medicaid.

In 1969, Mafia control of two New Jersey nursing homes was mentioned in tapes introduced in evidence in the trial of Simone DeCalvacante and in 1978 the Detroit boss, Joseph Zerilli, was found to be among the owners of a nursing home in Lake County, Michigan.

In 1973 the wise guys were caught trying to extend their control of certain union health plans to federal programs. Frank Fitzsimmons, then president of the

Teamsters, took time out to meet with three California mobsters while in Palm Springs to participate in Bob Hope's golf tournament. He gave them the go ahead for the creation of the American Health Maintenance Organization. Alan Dorfman, the Teamster's "consultant" was asked to work out the details.

This effort was related to a similar plan to set a up a Teamster's Union health plan with the People's Industrial Consultants. That project called for the establishment of twenty clinics throughout Illinois and Michigan under the name of Master Care Clinics. The FBI found the plan was being bankrolled by Anthony Accardo and friends.

These two efforts were tied together by Dorfman and his associates Peter Milano, Sam Sciortino, Dr. Bruce Frome, and others listed in the Bureau's files as being friends of Louis Rosanova. People's Industrial Consultants was hired to line up clients for the American Health Maintenance Organization in Los Angeles.

American Health was one of a number of prepaid health programs that began to flourish in California in the early 1970s. The impetus for the plans came from the state's governor, Ronald Reagan, and his health director, Earl Brian. Both saw prepaid plans as the solution to the state's escalating health bills.

Fifty-four contracts for prepaid health plans were awarded by the end of 1974. They had 252,000 medicaid beneficiaries enrolled and were being paid something like $82 million.

Prepaid plans were established for every member they enrolled, rather than plans on a fee-for-service basis. They enrolled thousands and then, to maximize their profits, did everything possible to limit service.

Chet Jones made it his business to investigate the health plans in California. He was trying to do his job. It cost him his health and everything he had.

Chet had been an investigator for the state's Department of Health for eleven years. He had worked first in the Department of Alcoholic Beverage Control, then with the Bureau of Consumer Affairs (the agency that licenses physicians), and finally served for seven years with the state's medical program.

His experience with the medicaid program began in 1967 when he was moved into the program as senior investigator. He was the first investigator hired to work up violations in the medical program and he developed the state's system for enforcing the department's rules.

In 1969 Jones was promoted to senior special investigator. He was placed in charge of investigations in the Los Angeles, San Bernardino, and San Diego regions with ten staff members under his control. In 1971, his staff was expanded to fifty and he was placed in charge of the entire southern California region.

The last time I saw him, two years later, he was a security guard for the May Company.

"Beginning in 1971," he told me, "we were under orders to send all complaints to the Bureau in Sacramento. We could not investigate them. But we discovered that the Bureau in Sacramento did not investigate them either.

"By 1972, we were getting literally hundreds of complaints. I met with my departmental superiors, Everett Chamberlin and Gerald Rolfes, and discussed this with them. I told them as strongly as I could that our failure to go ahead was hurting the program and reducing morale.

"About the same time, the *Los Angeles Times* ran a story on the scandal and I was given the go-ahead. That lasted five days. When I objected, they took the San Diego and San Bernardino offices away from me."

Because he questioned the state's inaction, Chet was accused of being disloyal. His scope of authority and responsibilities were continually eroded.

The *Los Angeles Times* discovered that the prepaid health plans were turning 3,000 percent profits. The state's auditor general agreed, finding that only 48 percent of the money being paid to the fifteen contractors they surveyed was being spent on patient services. The rest went for administrative expenses and profits.

Soon thereafter, the state attorney general was forced to sue one of the contractors when it failed to pay more than $2 million of its customers' bills. The contractor, National Prepaid Health Plan, Inc., was one of several tied to Alan Dorfman.

Finally, the stench got so great the state turned around.

In June of 1977, John Leeming was arrested in Detroit. At the time, Leeming was the millionaire owner of Titan Laboratories.

Leeming's fortune and troubles began in 1974. At that time, his lab was in trouble. "We weren't paying kickbacks," he said.

He learned what we had learned earlier.

"You pay kickbacks or you don't stay in business. About 99 percent of the business we did was payoff."

To raise capital, Leeming borrowed $5,000 from a loan shark. Unable to pay and concerned for his safety, he sought the protection of "Tony Jack" Giacalone, one of the kingpins of the mob in Detroit.

Giacalone, who ran Detroit's gambling and loan-shark rackets for almost a quarter of century, listened quietly to Leeming's request.

"Come with me," he said.

Together they went to a pay phone in a nearby restaurant.

Tony Jack dialed a number.

"Do you recognize my voice," he said.

When he had a response, he said, "Put the lab thing on the back burner. I'll take care of it."

With that Giacalone declared himself a partner in the lab. In 1979, he plead guilty to conspiring to extort money from Leeming. The best estimate is that he took $70,000 from the laboratory in two years.

Giacalone was sentenced to three years in prison. Leeming, who had turned state's evidence, was absorbed by the Bureau's witness protection plan.

By the fall of 1978, thirty-five states reported evidence indicating organized crime involvement in schemes to rip off medicare and medicaid. Every one of the thirty-five states told us they had found ties to nursing homes. Half had also found ties to pharmacies, laboratories, and clinics.

In September of 1975, Eugene Zipperstein and twelve of his associates were indicted for medicaid fraud. Four of those indicted were pharmacists. One was a doctor. The rest were administrators of his clinics, including one who was pretending to be a doctor.

Two years earlier, Zipperstein's father, Alan, one of the architects of the empire, had been shot seven times with a chrome plated .32-caliber automatic.

Five months later, Robert Fields, Zipperstein's partner, was gunned down.

Despite the fact that witnesses to Fields' murder said there were two assailants, investigators concluded both crimes had been committed by a young black man, William Hill. Hill was said to have been paid $5,000 for the two hits by his employer, Max Kaye, a 66-year-old dentist.

Zipperstein had attributed the murder of his partner to a syndicate trying to move in on their business. Police concluded the two murders were the result of a personal dispute between Fields and Kaye.

Zipperstein was said to have been murdered by mistake. Kaye died of an apparent heart attack before anyone could ask him.

Four more members of the Zipperstein empire would die within the next two years. One of these was Bharat Travedi. Travedi had been one of the subjects of our clinical laboratory investigation.

Travedi, like Kaye, was said to have died of an apparent heart attack. He was in his thirties. There was no autopsy. The death certificate was signed by a doctor at a medicaid clinic and the body was cremated. He was cooperating with authorities before his untimely death.

Another of the victims was William Guthrie. Guthrie, a 66-year-old physician, was one of those indicted with Eugene Zipperstein. He was also said to be cooperating with investigators.

On September 29, 1976, he was found dead. According to the authorities, he had committed suicide. If so, it was a determined effort. Guthrie's throat had been cut with a razor blade. He then managed to jump out of a window, falling nine floors to his death. In addition to being determined, he must also have been compulsive since he apparently took the time to replace the razor in his top dresser drawer before jumping.

In 1978, shortly before he was to go to prison, Eugene Zipperstein, heir to the Zipperstein-Fields empire, was stabbed. His neck was slashed and there were multiple stab wounds to his chest.

He told police, "I don't want to talk about it."

William Hill, the man convicted of killing Alan Zipperstein and Robert Fields seemed to agree. Though still claiming to be innocent some two years after his conviction, Hill refused to speculate. In an interview for CBS with Phil Walters, he said, "Twenty million will buy a lot. It will buy your death, my death, the cameraman's death, anybody's death. So we can take it from there, ya know. There's more to this than meets the eye."

"What are you worried about in here?" Phil asked.

"I've been worried here man. I've been worried right here in this cell. Not of the fact of going to the chair, but I got to sleep real light. And I know money talks."

There is good reason for Hill to worry.

Before his medicaid life, Robert Fields had owned a pawn shop. He had a long arrest record but no convictions under the name of Robert Festenstein.

Organized crime reports list him as the nephew of Joseph Epstein, a major player in the underworld. Epstein's bosses were said to be Anthony "Big Tuna"

Accardo and Paul "The Waiter" Ricca.

Accardo was also named, along with Santo Trafficante, by a federal grand jury in Florida in a 1981 health insurance fraud involving the Laborer's International Union. The scheme involved laundering money through a land development company to kickback to the principals: Accardo, Trafficante, and seven union officials.

A week after my meeting with Dr. Port, I called the office to check in. A follow-up meeting was scheduled within the hour.

"Oh, I'm so glad you called," the receptionist said.

"What happened?"

We had arranged with the GSA to have my New York phone calls forwarded to the committee when I was out. It rang on my brother's private line.

Staff had been instructed not to touch his phone when he was out. Somebody forgot. One of the secretaries picked up the phone with our standard acknowledgement, "Senate Committee."

The phone went dead.

A moment later the phone rang again. Not knowing what else to do the girl answered the phone, "Total Health Care Industries."

A man asked to speak to Mr. Clancey. When the girl asked who was calling, the caller hung up.

Under the circumstances I wasn't surprised when Dr. Port didn't show. I placed a call to his clinic and was told he was out.

With some frustration, we closed the investigation down and I returned to Washington. Before leaving, I called Wilson to tell him what happened.

"It happens," he said. "Sometimes worse. Be careful, these guys are for real."

I told him I already had a mother but I appreciated the thought.

"You remember the Keller thing?"

"Yes."

"Somebody but a bullet through the back of the good doctor's head."

I was stunned.

A few weeks earlier, George had invited me to sit in on one of the U.S. Attorney's stunts. They had a doctor they were trying to turn. The doctor had been caught stealing from the government, but he was small change. The U.S. Attorney wanted to work up the ladder.

For some reason, the doctor was recalcitrant. It was strange because normally a doctor will rat on his mother and give up his parking space before doing hard time.

To encourage him, Wilson arranged for an appearance before a grand jury. The physician's appearance was timed so that his employers, the Keller brothers, would see him brought before the jury in what appeared to be protective custody.

As expected, the physician took the fifth. But rather than dismiss him, Wilson kept him there the better part of two hours. Wilson asked him everything, from where he got his shoes to what he thought of the Yankees' chances.

Meanwhile, the Kellers sweated it out. I watched in the waiting room as they paced back and forth and whispered to each other.

Finally, the doctor was dismissed and one of the brothers was called. He took the fifth as well. But rather than ask him about the Yankees, Wilson asked where the money went.

Wilson's questions were precise and detailed, based on what we knew of their financial arrangements and the way the clinics operated. He asked about percentage arrangements with specific physicians, kickbacks with laboratories, pharmacies, and factors, leading the Kellers to wonder what the employee had said.

I thought it was quite a stunt. The physician, on hearing what had happened, became anxious to help. Others apparently were not as amused.

"Is he all right?"

"He's lucky to be alive."

Two weeks later we were preparing for hearing. I was on my way to my brother's home to meet a CBS reporter and his producer.

We arrived at the same time to find the door ajar.

Inside, we found the french doors in the back had been forced open. The chain was dangling. There were black smudges along the door frame.

I took a quick look around and called the police. All that appeared to be missing was a camera, some film, and notes from the New York investigation.

Twenty minutes later, two detectives arrived. They looked around and said it was strange.

"Any of our boys would have thrown the silver, that calculator, and the rest of that gear into a pillow case and gone out the front door like Santa Claus."

They called the fingerprint brigade to be sure, but none of us expected any additional evidence.

"Whoever broke in here was either a real amateur or a real pro," the cop said.

I didn't bother to tell him what we were working on.

That night Val joined me at my home in Maryland. We worked on completing a report for the committee and went to sleep late.

The events of the last few weeks played on my mind. I kept replaying scenes in my head. Finally, I dozed off.

I was awakened by my brother.

"We've got company."

He pointed toward the garage.

Since the age of eight when I began understudying Mickey Mantle, I have slept with a baseball bat by my bed. I picked it up and went for the front door.

Always helpful, my brother threw on the lights.

We saw someone run from the house, jump into a waiting pickup and speed away.

When the police arrived this time, they found no sign of an intruder – except for the gasoline can and a couple of rags left in the middle of the garage.

In the morning, we called the committee chairman and he called the FBI. We made copies and turned over duplicates of all the sensitive documents before proceeding with our hearing.

A few months later in New York, the U.S. Attorney was able to identify Joseph Pagano, a member of the Genovese family, with the mob's infiltration of the clinics. Pagano and his associates were said to have been using strong-arm tactics and death threats to extort money from the health centers.

Clinic owners were threatened with arson or beatings if they refused to make monthly payments to the mob. In return for these kickbacks, the gangsters provided "protection" from competition – a guarantee that no other center would be allowed to open within a twenty-block area.

Chapter Six
Care Gaps
———❦———

"This one is the goosiest thing you ever saw," said the man with the nylon stocking over his face. "But she's not good for more than $500 at a time."

The witness was reading from his "goose list." A goose is one step below a pigeon.

"This lady has always bought good. She wants a policy that pays for a rest home. She won't have anything else. Go to the back door."

As he spoke the crude cutouts in his mask began to wander. Within moments, most of his face was exposed. Further evidence that God has a sense of humor.

Sometimes it's hard to tell the difference between a con man and a salesman. This one was on the line. He was selling a worthless product – "medigap" insurance – and he knew it. Somewhere along the line – about the time he was indicted – he developed a conscience and decided confession was good for the soul. He was truly repentant, he said, and eager to testify to the sins of his past profession until he walked in and saw the twenty-five cameras waiting. I guess he expected a private booth with a curtain.

He had demanded a disguise so his neighbors wouldn't know what he'd been doing for a living. We had improvised a crude mask from a hastily borrowed stocking, making quick cutouts to allow for the eyes and mouth. What we hadn't anticipated was the fact that the cutouts would expand as the stocking went over his face. It looked now something like an Olympic weightlifter's tee-shirt.

"I'll be very honest with you, " he said. "The public is meant to be taken."

"What do you mean?" Pepper asked.

"What I mean by that is the public lies to us. We're salesmen and if you have any knowledge of selling anything you know when a person says he wants to think about it, they really don't want what you're selling. That's when you put the pressure on because he's lying to you, and you're going to lie right back to him. It's a game."

"Why did your company pick on senior citizens?"

"They're easier to sell. Probably 50 percent of the time they are widows or widowers. They are alone. So you only have to convince one person."

"And these are the people you have been describing on your list?"

"Some of them. "

"Some of them?"

"These are repeaters. They'll buy anything, if you know how to come at them. Here's another one. She's easy. But you've got to make the right pitch. The note says she's worried about her sister. Be sure to talk about cancer coverage and tell her that pre-existing conditions are covered."

"So it's what some people would call a sucker list."

"You could say that."

"How long did it take you to develop that list?"

"Twenty years. I bought a starter. But I've added to it over the last twenty years. "

"You bought a starter?"

"Right. Salesmen sell their lists or trade them to each other."

"How much do they go for?"

"I paid $5,000. They go for more now. Depending on how many names are on the list."

"Have you ever sold that list?"

"Yes."

"What did you get?"

"Twelve grand, the last time."

More than three-fourths of the elderly have some form of supplemental insurance coverage. The rest harbor the mistaken belief that medicare and medicaid provide comprehensive service.

Sitting behind the salesman was the son of one of his victims. He too had expressed concern for potential embarrassment. He asked that his mother not be identified.

"I'm here to tell you my mother was sold an unbelievable seventy-one insurance policies," he told the committee.

His 76-year-old mother lived alone on the family farm in southern Illinois. The farm, purchased on a forty-year mortgage, had been paid off two years earlier.

"Her annual income from the farm is $9,400. This income is sufficient for her needs since she lives a simple life. However, in the past three years, since our father's death, she has accumulated a debt of $3,000, which has been generated by the payment of insurance premiums."

Total payments in the last year had exceeded $15,000 and were sufficient to force the widow to refinance the farm.

When we discovered this fact, her first reaction was to defend the agents. "I know they wouldn't sell me anything I didn't need," she said. "They are just trying to protect me from the huge medical and hospitals bills I might have later on."

After the death of her husband, the salesman had established a close relationship with the widow. He was the same age as her children. After a while, she almost came to think of him as a member of the family.

They thought of her as an easy mark, a "goose."

If it was any consolation, she now knew she wasn't alone. She was one of thousands who were being victimized by salesmen who had been trained to prey on the fact that twenty-five years after medicare was enacted, access to health care remains seniors' primary concern.

Like a number of others, this investigation had been triggered by a letter.

"Last spring, I learned my 88-year-old aunt whose annual income is less than $5,000 had been sold more than $10,400 of health insurance in approximately a year's time," the author wrote.

The policies and copies of the cancelled checks were enclosed. The checks were good. The policies were not. They were duplicative, cancelling each other out. She was no more insured with ten than she was with one.

All she received for her money was indemnification for the deductible and co-insurance amounts medicare required beneficiaries to pay – at most a few hundred dollars.

A survey of the states, which have the primary responsibility for regulating insurance companies, turned up a series of related stories. The Tennessee Department of Insurance reported a company that paid back less than thirty-three cents on the dollar in claims. The average among reputable companies is around seventy-five cents on the dollar.

The company in question advertised it paid up to $300 per operation. The only way you could collect that much was to have cranial brain surgery, which would cost at least $1,500.

The Commissioner of Insurance in North Carolina reported instances in which elderly consumers were sold "replacement" policies every four months, causing the old policy to lapse and generating extra income for the salesmen.

In New Jersey, three agents from the same company sold a woman eleven policies: five hospital indemnity policies, three nursing home policies, and three medicare supplemental policies.

Other states reported salesmen who posed as representatives of social security, salesmen claiming to represent the victim's accident and health insurance company, salesmen claiming to be engaged in surveys of seniors' needs, salesmen representing radio and television advertisements offering information for the elderly, and appeals by high-priced shills.

A "fact book" bearing Paul Harvey's name was a popular entry gimmick for a while. Now they're using Dick Van Dyke, Gavin MacLeod, Lorne Greene, Tennessee Ernie Ford, and, of course, Ed McMahon.

The worst are the "dread disease" policies.

Playing on fears of cancer and other dread diseases, some of the smaller, less reputable insurance companies have carved out a nice little niche for themselves. By misrepresenting the risk of the disease and overstating the benefit of their policies, they were among the fastest growing and most profitable companies in the United States.

We recruited a friend of Congressman Pepper's, Margaret Dixon, to help us document the problem. Margaret said she had always wanted to be an actress and thought she could be as "goosy" as the next person. She was placed on the committee's payroll as a consultant.

Margaret made a series of random calls to insurance companies offering health insurance. When the salesmen arrived, she showed them her standard Blue Cross policy and asked if she needed any additional coverage.

In the corner of her living room, a somewhat large, somewhat hairy apparition who looked something like my brother, sat playing with a Nikon draped around his neck. He seemed totally preoccupied with the $500 toy.

Occasionally, he grimaced and uttered some inarticulate sound out of a contorted face.

"He's handicapped," Margaret explained. "He's always been like that."

The salesmen invariably averted their eyes.

Generally about that time, my brother would focus and fire off a couple of frames.

"Not to worry," she said. "There's no film in there. We just let him play with it to keep him quiet."

Fifty salesmen in nine states and the District of Columbia stopped by to make their pitch and be photographed. Eight of them were ethical.

The others demonstrated how creative an average, high-school educated American can be when properly motivated.

In California, a "twister" advised Margaret to drop her AARP policy, saying it was no good. He tried to sell her three other policies.

One of the New York sharpies told Margaret she needed six different policies from three companies. He offered everything from a "hospital benefit plan" to cancer care and a burial plan. He hadn't bothered to examine her existing insurance before making his suggestions. "They're all worthless," he said.

Others presented documents, credentials, and policies designed to look like they were issued by the government; misrepresented the contents and cost of their policies; quoted weekly rates for annual policies; invited us to "make the check out to me" or post-date applications; and switched policies, substituting a more expensive policy for the one described at the close.

The most common abuse was "overloading." The vast majority of salesmen who came through our door tried to sell Margaret more insurance than she needed.

The second most prevalent abuse is called "clean sheeting." The salesmen promised us "better coverage" by "ignoring" Margaret's pre-existing health conditions. If Margaret had ever tried to collect on these policies, her claims would have been rejected and she would have been accused of trying to defraud the insurer by claiming to be in good health.

In Philadelphia, a salesman took the direct approach. The first question he asked was, "How much of your weekly income can you spare?"

In the District of Columbia, an unusually energetic con man who looked like he could commit any crime that did not require courage concluded his pitch by asking Margaret for her power of attorney.

We concluded one out of every four dollars spent annually for supplemental policies was being wasted. The rip-off factor was estimated at $3 billion.

Ethel Hurst, an 88-year-old woman, is one of those who was fleeced. Terrified that long-term illness would bankrupt her, she bought twenty-eight medigap policies. But when she fractured her hip and had a mastectomy, her nephew found out the policies were worthless. The $5,500 she had spent to purchase protection might as well have been stolen.

A 76-year-old North Carolina woman was another victim. She was frightened into buying thirteen supplemental policies in two years. The premiums amounted to half of her total income.

An analysis of cancer and other dread disease policies indicated they are practically worthless. They provide little additional benefit to consumers while generating enormous profit to the insurance companies. Typically, they keep sixty to eighty cents of every premium dollar for themselves. A slot machine offers better odds.

By comparison, the average for health insurance companies nationally is a return of 80 percent – eighty cents of every dollar collected in insurance premiums returned to the insured in payment of claims.

Pepper, the venerable champion of the elderly, was outraged. He said these "medigyp policies" posed "a national scandal of staggering dimensions."

The worst of it is that many of the fears that drive seniors to buy these policies are justified. But there is no policy or combination of policies they can buy that will plug up medicare and medicaid's gaping holes.

There is a profound and bitter irony in the fact that more than twenty-five years after the enactment of medicare and medicaid, and despite the expenditure of billions of dollars, seniors still spend as much of their out-of-pocket income for health care as they did in 1965 before these programs were enacted.

From the beginning, the medicare/medicaid debate focused on the question of who, not what. Who would pay for the services? Who would deliver the care? Who would be eligible to receive the services provided?

As a result, we have a system unlike any other in the world.

Every other developed nation, with the exception of South Africa, provides comprehensive insurance for all of their citizens. We provide selected services to all seniors and some services to some of the poor – though half of those with an income under $11,000 are ineligible for medicaid.

Every other nation has organized their health care so that the majority of services are delivered as close to the patients' residences as possible. We have a system that emphasizes institutionalization.

Other nations emphasize early intervention, home care, and hospice. Medicare, the largest federal program, will not provide service unless the patient is acutely ill and has some hope of recovery.

Neither medicare, medicaid, the Veterans Administration, nor any other state or federal program will pay for preventative services, even though it is better medicine and has long been proven to be cost-effective. The cost-effectiveness of prevention to treatment has been estimated to be sixteen to one ever since the days of Benjamin Franklin.

Other countries consolidate sophisticated services requiring high technology in regional health centers. We make even the most expensive equipment available to every six-bed county medical center.

In all, medicare pays less than half of the medical bills for the elderly. No provision was made for payment of dental services, eyeglasses, eye examinations, hearing care, preventative care, foot care, or long-term care.

Nor was the question of the kind of care ever broadly debated. Scarce attention was paid to the matter of quality assurance, other than the medical community's insistence that something other than full payment of their prevailing rate would assure poor care.

The fact of the matter is that we do not have a health system. Rather, we have many health systems. We have one system for the elderly. Another for the poor. A third for the nine million military servicemen on active duty. A fourth for veterans. A fifth for native Americans. And yet another for those who can afford to pay. Within the private sector there are just as many subcategories, based on how much one can afford to pay for what.

For many Americans, there is no system at all. Over fifty million Americans are entirely without health insurance.

Henry Valdez is one of those who fell between the cracks. My brother found him living in a chicken coop in New Mexico.

He was 70 years old. The chicken coop was provided by the city.

Henry was one of thousands of mentally ill people who were dumped into the streets beginning in the early 1970s.

So was Alice Jackson.

Alice was born in 1873 when Rutherford B. Hayes was president. She had been a concert pianist, a Ziegfield showgirl, a journalist, and had helped manage the gubernatorial and presidential campaigns of Al Smith and Franklin D. Roosevelt.

There were over 400,000 people in state hospitals on an average day in 1969. Only 200,000 remained by the end of 1975.

Many of these people were elderly. All of them were ill. Though there was talk of community placement and service, little was provided. Today, the mentally ill line the streets of every metropolitan city.

Like so many others, this trend began in California. In 1966 then Governor Ronald Reagan announced a policy designed to remove the state completely from providing care to the mentally ill.

By the end of 1974 the number of patients in state hospitals had been reduced from over 30,000 to 6,476. The number of elderly in these hospitals was reduced by 95 percent.

One of those released was Charles Soper. Within months of his release, Soper took a .22-caliber rifle and killed his wife, their three children, and himself. The state had certified he "no longer presented a danger to himself or others" before releasing him. The state was wrong.

John Phillip Bunyard, released after sixteen years in an asylum, told the court, "I don't want to go out there. I feel like a puppy you are putting on the freeway. I don't think I can make it."

Bunyard committed two murders, two rapes, and several kidnappings before he was captured.

New York followed California. In the first ten years, the number of patients in New York state hospitals was reduced from 75,000 to about 25,000. Currently, it is estimated that there are only 4,000 patients in New York's mental hospitals.

Patients were discharged wholesale and indiscriminately. Almost overnight, psychiatric ghettos developed across the country and the "homeless" were born. Between 40 and 60 percent of the homeless are former mental patients or are mentally ill.

With the mentally ill, progress is measured slowly. They are among the millions in this country who require long-term care.

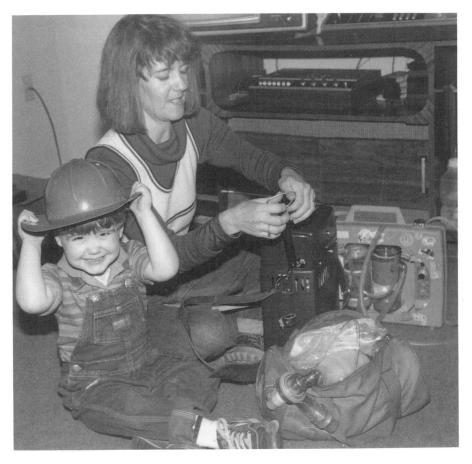

photo by Marilu Halamandaris
Jeff Reckeweg with his home care nurse. Born with a rare disease known as Ondine's Curse, Jeff is one of nearly 10 million children in this country who need long-term care.

Alex Sutton is another.

Four-year-old Alex is a victim of Tay-Sachs disease. When he was about a year old, his development began to reverse.

"At the time, they were telling us he would live, maybe, five years," his mother said. "They said his development would reverse and he'd go back to being a baby, which is pretty much where he is now."

Because Alex's condition was not going to improve, no financial assistance was available for the Suttons.

Nor is there any assistance for Peter Fiterman, Katherine Fischer, Danny Russell, or Jeff Reckeweg.

Peter was in a motorcycle accident his sophomore year at Tulane. His family had a $600,000 medical insurance policy. That money was gone within thirteen months. "I never dreamed this could happen," Mrs. Fiterman said. "We have been devastated. I don't know what I can say to you except something is wrong when a family can be annihilated from an illness like this."

Katherine Fischer was born with a chromosone defect. She couldn't hear or speak. She suffered from heart, kidney, and intestinal ailments. The Fischers took care of their daughter around the clock for fifteen years without asking for the assistance they were entitled to under their insurance policy. When the burden became too great and they requested assistance, the policy was changed.

Danny Russell was born prematurely. His lungs had not fully developed. He needs assistance breathing. The State of Michigan said it would provide that assistance but only if he stays in a hospital.

"You're really faced with a choice of leaving your child in the hospital where all the bills are paid," Mrs. Russell said, "or bringing him home, knowing that it's better for your child and better for your family – and paying for it out of pocket, if you can, and paying for the insurance besides."

For some the choice is even more inhumane.

"Practically the only option if you live in Arizona is to make your child a ward of the state," Mrs. Sutton said. "But he's our baby. We don't want to give him up. They even have the option to place your child in someone else's home if they want to."

The cost of caring for Alex was over $250,000 a year.

There are now over ten million children in this country who are chronically ill. Over the last twenty-five years they have increased from 2 percent to 4 percent of all children. Because of the progress of technology, which can save children who, earlier, might have died, that number will double again by the end of the century.

The choices faced by families with chronically ill children are not unlike the choices given adults with chronically ill parents.

Marion Roach, the daughter of an Alzheimer's Disease victim told us, "My doctor advised me that the only way to get financial assistance for my mother would be to break her arm, and have her put in a hospital."

"He said when her arm heals, break it again, and keep breaking it if you want to be assured of financial assistance."

Medicare is structured to underwrite treatment of diseases that can be cured. There is no treatment for Alzheimer's Disease, no cure for chronic conditions.

Medicaid was designed for the poor, though one must be increasingly poor to apply. There is no assistance whatsoever for the middle class. "We took out a mortgage on the house and rent a small apartment for my mother," Mrs. Roach said. "She now lives there with round-the-clock home care. It is costing us $4,000 a month. At that rate, we will be completely broke in two years."

The only viable alternative, nursing home placement , would have been twice as expensive.

There is another remedy, but not one I would recommend.

Johanna Florian, a 52-year-old south Florida woman, also developed Alzheimer's Disease. After caring for her devotedly for six years, Ralph Florian, her husband, nineteen years older and himself in poor health, shot and killed her.

All of the excesses or our health system and most of our expenditures have been directed at acute conditions that require hospitalization. Medicare's rule has been: If we can treat it and the patient will get better, we will pay for it. Otherwise, we will not.

The number of people in this country with chronic diseases that require long-term care is escalating dramatically. In part this is because of our success in treating acute conditions, but largely it is a result of demographics. We face a staggering challenge.

A quarter of our population will be over sixty-five by the year 2000. Eighteen percent of all people over the age of sixty-five have chronic health conditions that prevent them from carrying out normal activities.

Nine million of these will be veterans whom we are obligated to care for through the Veterans Administration. There were 3.3 million veterans over sixty-five in 1981.

Ninety percent of nursing home residents are over sixty-five. There were about one million people in nursing homes in 1980. There will be twice as many in the year 2000, and five million by 2050.

Seven out of ten will be impoverished within thirteen weeks of their entry into a nursing home. As it is, the cost of caring for catastrophic long-term care forces more than a million Americans into poverty each year.

Add the AIDS population to these.

There are currently 1.5 million people – predominantly young adults – who carry the AIDS virus. Most of them will develop the disease. The number of active cases will triple within three years – from 50,000 to 270,000 – and continue to increase progressively from there.

Before the turn of the century, AIDS will be one of the leading cases of death in America and the leading cause of death among people aged twenty-five to forty-four. It is estimated that we are currently spending about $15 billion to care for AIDS victims. It is expected that total will triple by the year 2000.

The nature of the care they need, like the care required by chronically ill children and seniors, is low-tech and long-term. AIDS victims, like the kids and seniors, will find there is currently no federal or state program that will provide significant assistance.

Chapter Seven
Paper Doctors
—— ❦ ——

"I can give to you an M.D.," Pedro said.

He was in his mid-sixties, tall, and distinguished.

"Who is going to sponsor your medical career?"

"I guess I'll have to get a loan. How much will it be?"

"Usually in matters like this, it is over $20,000," Pedro said. "But I will be able to do some special price for you."

"How special?"

"I think I will be able to charge you $16,500 – from which I need $5,600 with the application before you go to take your degree."

"Save time, save money," the ad in the *Washington Post* had read. Several hundred people had answered that ad. One hundred and sixty-four came up with the money. One hundred and sixty-three were not investigators.

When Pedro said "take your degree" he was being literal. No formal schooling was involved. The only requirement for matriculation was cash or adequate credit.

"I'm doing something special for you," Pedro said, "because I have sympathy for you."

He sounded sincere.

"You will remember me for the rest of your life. Perhaps you will take care of my grandchildren and my children free."

In October, Pedro and the future physician met again. "You are scheduled to graduate in December, right?"

The investigator had not left the country since first talking to Pedro and had never been to Santo Domingo, where his medical degree would be issued.

"That's right."

"You have to go to this place."

"Why?"

"For examination."

"I wasn't aware I would have to take an examination."

"You have to do it. But this is a formality."

"Are the tests fairly easy to pass?"

"You don't care you pass or not. You will have no problem."

"So far as the university is concerned, my transcripts and everything will be okay but will FLEX accept them?"

FLEX is the Federation Licensing Examination. It is administered by the states as part of the medical licensing process.

"FLEX will not create you any problems," Pedro said.

He was right. By the time the authorities caught up with him, forty of his clients had been certified by the Educational Commission for Foreign Medical Graduates. Thirteen had obtained their medical licenses and six more were working in hospital residency programs.

We went up to see him after he was sentenced. They had sent him to the Allenwood "Country Club" and Correctional Center in Pennsylvania.

They'd nailed Pedro for mail fraud and sentenced him to three years of not-so-hard time. Part of his sentence was an agreement to cooperate with federal officials trying to undo what he had done.

Pedro thought the sentence was harsh. After all, he hadn't committed much of a crime. In his mind, it was something of a public service. "It is extremely difficult to obtain admission to American medical schools," he said. "You have to be very bright. You have to have a 3.7 or a 3.8 just to get an interview. And it is very expensive. The average person cannot become a doctor in America."

Pedro made it easy for them. He also made a piece of change. He admitted a take in excess of $1.5 million in three years.

We had backed into this one. But we should have seen it coming. It was predictable, given the evolution of what we had begun calling Medigate.

In medicaid's first year, a paper doctor named Warren Slough was arrested for performing an abortion on a Brooklyn college student. Fifteen years later, he would be arrested again on similar charges. In the interim, though he continued his practice, he still hadn't found the time to go to medical school.

A few years earlier, Shelly Styles had confessed to us that his first medicaid experience was to pose as the senile Dr. Portoguese to run up the government's tab. Through the years, we had run into similar cases in New York, Pennsylvania, and California.

Half of the people we interviewed in the Chicago storefront clinic we had opened as a test a decade before Pedro came along held foreign medical degrees. The Illinois Office of Special Investigations pulled hundreds of their records and concluded there was "significant evidence" that some of these individuals lacked basic training. Others were said to have doctored their files and resorted to payoffs.

A few years later, Anthony Struich of Cleveland admitted he had falsely received $48,000 from the government by posing as a physician. About the same time, a janitor for a Miami clinic was arrested for pretending to be a physical therapist.

If that wasn't enough, we had the testimony of one of the welfare doctors we had interviewed in depth prior to sentencing. He had every reason to be forthcoming and was. "The only time the doctor sees a patient in one of these places," he said, "is when the patient walks by him either to the lab or the pharmacy. The patient is usually served by unlicensed physicians – immigrants who may or may not have a license."

Despite the evidence, we probably still would not have connected the dots had it not been for Max.

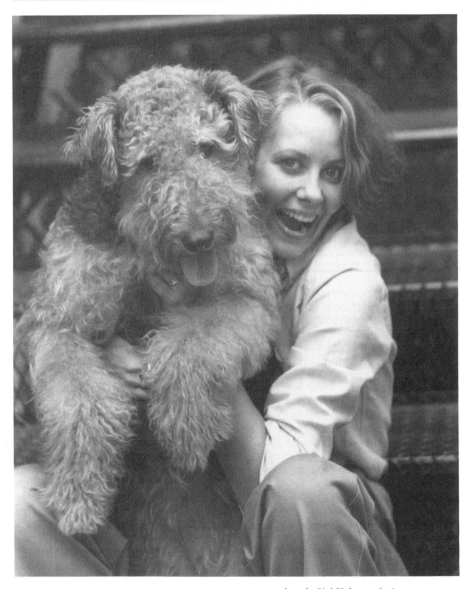

photo by Val Halamandaris
*The Rev. Dr. B. B. Maxwell, M.D., J.D., Ph.D., A.K.C.,
and friend.*

The Reverend B. B. Maxwell is truly remarkable. She is a minister, licensed to preach the gospel in California. She is a physician, a lawyer, has a Ph.D., and is listed in several indices of outstanding Americans.

All and all, that's not bad for an Airedale.

By accident I had found myself thumbing through the advertisements in one of our more disreputable periodicals one morning. Like everyone else, I don't read those things except when standing in line at the supermarket where one has no choice.

As I waited to be scanned, my eyes fixed on an interesting advertisement. For a token amount, the ad said, one could be credentialed in any field of choice.

I found myself wondering what you would get if you responded to one these implausible ads, if there was any credibility to their claims and, if not, how they got away with what they said.

Since Val and I already have several degrees we don't use, I decided I'd get one for Max. She has always been shy around strangers. I thought a college degree – perhaps a doctor of divinity – might help her self-image.

I put a money order for twenty-five dollars in the mail (Max didn't have a checking account at the time). Within two weeks a diploma suitable for framing arrived. It looked as good as mine and was probably more valuable since it came with instructions on how to set up your own church. The brochure touted the advantages of being your own boss and carefully noted there were some significant tax advantages.

That made sense to me. Max agreed.

In short order, Max was getting more mail than I was. She seemed to be on every mailing list in the country. She received solicitations for everything from self-study courses in the martial arts to mail-order brides from Europe, Japan, and the Philippines.

A distressing amount of the material was pitched at the poor and elderly – everything from phoney business schemes to home-grown health remedies. These we began to catalogue and take seriously. The poor were a prime target for business frauds. The elderly were most susceptible to health frauds. Poor seniors get a double whammy, constituting about 30 percent of all fraud victims.

With the help of investigators detailed by the U.S. Postal Service, we began a systematic collection of suspicious ads, clipping every newspaper and magazine on the racks. We found more rackets than you would believe possible. By the time we were done, we had volumes of reports and had conducted hearings on fraudulent work-at-home schemes, investment schemes, get-rich-quick schemes, home repair games, and quackery.

All of it was bad and blatant. But the health frauds were most troublesome. The advertisements preyed on the fears and desperation of the sick and dying. Their success was fueled by the growing cost of medical care and the elderly's growing disenchantment with the medical profession.

Over a four-year period, we documented some truly outrageous scams. Distilled water, seaweed extracts, ground diamonds, mistletoe extracts drawn at the time of the full moon, ground warts from horses, serums distilled from fecal matter, urine, and the like were touted as cures for cancer.

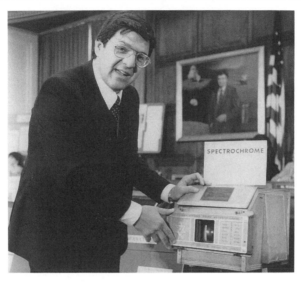

photo by Marilu Halamandaris
Val with the Spectrochrome. Touted as a cure for everything from cancer to arthritis, the Spectrochrome was nothing more than a metal box with a lightbulb at its center.

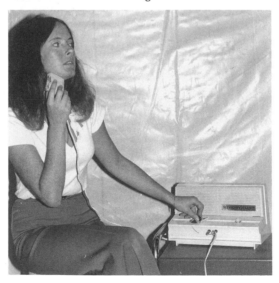

photo by Val Halamandaris
Kathy Garnder with a quack device known as a "revitilizer."

Arthritics were promised relief from "cures" composed of venom from snakes and ants, diets of honey and herbs, and extracts of plants, pepper, and parsley. The patient sufferers were advised to sit in abandoned mine shafts, bury themselves in warm manure, bathe in kerosene and cod liver oil, and stand naked under a 1,000 watt lamp at the time of the full moon.

The samples we gathered were reviewed by a panel of sixty national experts. None of the products we had obtained by mail did what they claimed. About 75 percent were found to be harmful.

Some of the products contained narcotics. Others were contaminated and could have caused death. Many offered dangerous advice – like looking directly into the sun to cure glaucoma.

We concluded quackery had become big business. The committee estimated something in excess of $10 billion a year was being ripped off by the purveyors of these worthless products.

Pedro upped the ante.

Pedro said he had been a member of an advisory council for the president of the United States and had served as an advisor to a cabinet committee created by Nixon to help Hispanic minorities. He had engaged in this scheme with every intention of continuing his public service. He said he hoped to gather enough money to run for president of Peru.

In the three years he was in business, Pedro provided false transcripts for about one hundred clients. The transcripts indicated these "students" had fulfilled the medical requirements of schools they hadn't attended. He also arranged placements in American schools for clinical rotations and falsified evaluations of clinical rotations.

In both cases, the key was money.

Pedro said he only got to keep a third of the money he collected. The rest went for "tuition" payments, gifts to assistant deans, and miscellaneous expenses associated with administering tests to student who are not present.

One of Pedro's beneficiaries was an American with a degree in hospital administration from Columbia and a medical degree as a neurosurgeon from Loyola. "This is the dean who handed me the fake documents," Pedro said. "He wiped out the names on transcripts belonging to bona fide students who applied to the school and told me, 'You just type the name there. Make sure your students go to a notary and notarize their signature. Then return the documents to me.'"

One of those was a pharmacist named Harry Lee. In one year and for less than ten thousand dollars, Lee was able to gain admittance to a foreign medical school without taking the MCAT, without legitimate recommendations, with a "C" grade point average, and without any knowledge of Spanish.

While Lee got a degree from a medical school without ever going to class, he did have to do clinical rotations. Lee went to Polk General Hospital in Florida, for three and a half weeks. He subsequently took and passed the equivalency exam for foreign medical graduates and would have been practicing medicine today if Pedro hadn't made a misstep.

About 21 percent of all licensed physicians are foreign medical graduates. While there are over 1,000 foreign medical schools, the many of those who practice in the United States come from a few "border" colleges.

Over one third of all foreign medical graduates come from Central and South America and the vast majority of American citizens studying abroad can be found in less than a dozen schools. Three schools enroll 50 percent of U.S. citizens studying medicine abroad.

All of these schools were established subsequent to the enactment of medicare and medicaid. Most of them were established after 1970 when the profitability of public medicine was assured.

In 1980 the General Accounting Office reviewed the operation of six of these foreign medical schools and concluded that none of them offered a medical education comparable to that available in the United States. Deficiencies in admission requirements (some had admitted people without high school degrees), curriculums, faculty, and clinical training were noted. Most rudimentary equipment, such as x-ray machines, research libraries, and patients was lacking.

Because of the high public esteem and enviable financial rewards associated with the practice of medicine, many more Americans want to become doctors than can be accommodated in American schools, despite the fact that the number of American medical students has doubled in the last twenty years.

Since medicare's enactment, the nation's physician supply has risen 70 percent. Pre-medicare, the average number of annual medical school graduates was about 7,000. Today, it exceeds 17,000.

Despite this increase, only half of those who apply to American medical schools are accepted. Many of the rest, some 15,000, apply to foreign schools as a last resort.

Many of these schools are more interested in obtaining American dollars than they are in training competent physicians. At the time of Pedro's incarceration, Americans spent $50 million for medical tuition and living expenses in the Dominican Republic. The dozen medical schools in that nation of six million form one of the most profitable industries in the country.

Americans pay up to $2,500 per trimester to attend these schools – or rather their government pays for them, since most of these students benefit from federal or state educational loans (to the tune of $45 million in 1982). Locals pay $75. With that kind of differential, it shouldn't be a surprise if their admission standards for Americans are flexible.

The second step down the yellow brick road is participation in undergraduate clinical training programs. Most of the foreign medical schools patronized by Americans do not have the capacity to provide clinical training. They rely instead on arrangements for placement in the United States.

Dr. Joseph McPike, formerly of Polk General Hospital in Bartow, Florida, was one of those who helped arrange these rotations. He was indicted and convicted of stealing more than $20,000 that students had paid for clinical training.

What about competency tests and professional licensing requirements?

Before foreign medical graduates can practice in the United States they have to pass two tests: an examination by the Educational Commission for Foreign Medical

Graduates (ECFMG), a private testing organization, and the Federation Licensing Examination, administered by the state in which the applicant wants to be licensed.

In July of 1983, 17,000 students took the ECFMG examination. Three to four thousand of these applicants were found to have obtained the questions and correct answers in advance. Someone had bought a copy of the test for $50,000. The purchaser, demonstrating his aptitude for medicine, made multiple copies and sold them for $25,000 each. These purchasers made copies which sold for $10,000. The chain letter process continued until, ultimately, copies were available for $50.

Similarly, cheating has been documented in the licensing examinations of the majority of states and for those less risk-oriented, there is always public service. The federal government does not require its physicians to be licensed. Fifty percent of all foreign medical graduates receive training in facilities run by the Veterans Administration.

Stephen Berger claimed to be a graduate of CETEC, one of Pedro's Caribbean colleges. In fact, he had only attended two of ten required semesters. Nevertheless, he entered the army as a first lieutenant in 1981. He worked at the Irwin Army Hospital at Fort Riley for a year and then began a four-year residency at Letterman Army Medical Center in San Francisco. From 1982 to 1984, he spent half of each week in surgery, performing amputations, hip replacements, and complicated hand operations.

When Berger was discovered, the army's excuse was that it had relied on the Educational Commission for Foreign Medical Graduates to validate foreign medical degrees.

Abraham Assante posed as a physician for almost fifteen years. He worked in a number of hospitals in New York and rose to the position of Chief Medical Officer in the military. He even managed to obtain a fellowship to the National Institute of Health where he worked for six months before being dismissed.

In 1983, Assante was employed as a staff anaesthesiologist at Watson Army Hospital in Fort Dix when Joseph Branda came in for a routine operation. Branda was forty-seven years old. He had been in the military for twenty years, was in excellent health, and had recently been married. He was told the procedure would last fifteen minutes.

During the operation, Branda's heart stopped. According to hospital records, Assante did not notice for four minutes. By the time Branda's heart could be started, he had suffered irreparable brain damage. He will need round-the-clock nursing care for the rest of his life.

Pedro's arrest and the subsequent attempt to identify and find individuals who had purchased degrees led to what came to be called the "largest medical scandal in recent medical history." Criminal investigations were initiated in fifteen states. The process by which foreign medical graduates are licensed in the United States and the quality of education provided by these foreign medical schools was brought into question.

In short order, other brokers were identified and placed under investigation. In all, credentials of some ten thousand practicing physicians were questioned.

How is it possible that these paper doctors could continue to practice undetected for years?

Primary responsibility for regulating physicians and monitoring their professional performance has traditionally rested with the states. Our experience with the state licensing process is not encouraging.

In the first ten years of the medicare and medicaid programs, the State of New York received fifty-three cases of alleged professional misconduct. We found the City of New York had suspended or disqualified 120 practitioners from medicaid alone during that period and sixty-six of these had been referred for criminal action.

Of the fifty-three cases referred for criminal action, the state took action in five cases. New York has a reputation for having one of the better licensing programs in the nation.

The activities of state medical boards are nationally coordinated by a federation formed three-quarters of a century ago. In 1984, the federation reported the states had collectively disciplined 1,389 of the nation's 430,000 physicians.

That total represents a fraction (one out of every 252) of the doctors involved in malpractice settlements in that year. It must also be placed in the context of the American Medical Association's estimates that 10,000 doctors are alcoholics and that another 4,000 are drug addicts.

On average, the states discipline less than 1 percent of all physicians a year. They seem to see their role as being confined to issuing and renewing licenses. There is no appetite for investigation and examination.

Maryland's experience is typical. In 1987, Maryland's Commission on Medical Discipline received 862 complaints against doctors. They held four hearings and revoked one license.

Three-quarters of the physicians the state has disciplined over the last twenty years were put on probation. They include thirty-five doctors who were convicted of sex crimes, drug charges, theft, and medicaid fraud.

One of these people, a Baltimore gynecologist, was convicted of raping a patient. Another, a psychiatrist, was convicted of repeated medicaid fraud and drug abuse.

In a third case, a family practitioner was convicted of assault. The court found the physician had gone to a woman's home, drugged her, and assaulted her. After reviewing the evidence, the licensing commission concluded the doctor's practice did not conform with "acceptable therapeutic regimes" and put him on probation for three years.

What happens to a doctor who happens to be so unfortunate as to be caught and disciplined?

The General Accounting Office reviewed records in three states. They found that thirty-three of 181 doctors who had been disciplined simply moved elsewhere and continued their practice.

In a follow-up investigation, the Department of Health and Human Services found 271 doctors who continued their practice and billed the government for their services even though their licenses had been revoked. Collectively, these doctors had received $8.5 million in three years from medicare and another $338,400 from medicaid.

By the end of 1985, investigators had identified another 1,000 phoney medical practitioners. One of them killed Alma Agnis.

Alma went into a Las Vegas clinic for cosmetic surgery. She was forty-two. She wanted breast augmentation and stretch marks removed from her stomach.

Unfortunately, her "doctor" was really an accountant and chiropractor with delusions of grandeur. He didn't know that the three narcotics he gave Alma were deadly in combination. Investigators discovered the chiropractor was on probation in California where he had been previously convicted three times of practicing medicine without a license.

By this time, we had returned to where we started. It was clear the problem of phoney credentials was not limited to the medical community. The FBI joined in and with an operation they called "Dipscam," identified thousands of phoney doctors, chiropractors, psychiatrists, engineers, teachers, and other professionals. One of their cases, an Oregon diploma mill, had conferred phoney degrees on 2,300 customers.

Another of the Bureau's finds was an enterprising individual named Anthony Geruntino. Geruntino had sold 3,000 diplomas attributed to various universities through his post office box. Two hundred of these diplomas were sold to federal employees. Another two hundred went to people employed by state governments.

In the aggregate, it is now said that half a million Americans are hiding behind paper credentials.

What about Max?

Not long ago, she received an invitation to join the International Platform Speakers Association. The association bills itself with some justification as "one of the most prestigious and influential organizations in the United States." The solicitation was kind enough to point out that this honor was not offered to everyone and that an acceptance would put Max in the company of some of our most distinguished Americans. Former President Ronald Reagan is a member. So are Richard Nixon, Malcom Forbes, Barbara Walters, Harry Truman, Robert Novak, and Patrick Buchanan, to name a few.

Understandably, Max was honored. I agreed and encouraged her to join. I figure Max has as much to say as any of them.

Chapter Eight
Pumping Gold

———— 🂠 ————

"Let me tell you a little bit about the way we work."

We were in the psychiatric ward of a hospital in Brooklyn borrowed for the occasion. The speaker was a salesman who made more than a million dollars a year.

"All of our equipment is offered totally free of charge."

He placed a half dozen pieces of electronic equipment on the desk between us and began to itemize.

"We wouldn't charge you for transmitters."

Transmitters are used to monitor a pacemaker's performance. They sell for about two to three hundred dollars each.

"That's one per person, right?"

"We'll give you dozens. We'll send dozens."

"What about a receiver?"

Receivers catch the transmitters' signals. They sell for three to four thousand dollars.

"You can have five receivers if you need them."

We were nearing the conclusion of an investigation of the pacemaker industry. The investigation had begun more than a year before when an eighty-eight-year-old woman, Madeline Garman, wrote the committee an angry letter.

"You may not be the ones to handle this problem," she said. "If not, you will know whom to give it to."

Mrs. Garman, a nurse and social worker, had just had surgery to replace a defective pacemaker.

Despite the fact that the pacemaker had been guaranteed and that eight years remained on the warranty, medicare had been charged for the replacement. Mrs. Garman asked, why?

In all, medicare had paid more than $12,000 for her two pacemaker operations in less than two years.

"How many hundreds of these were recalled over the country and how many thousands of dollars were spent by medicare?" she queried. "It is one of the ways medicare is being milked, and I am sick of it."

"When a car is recalled, there is no expense to the customer. Why should medicare pay this?"

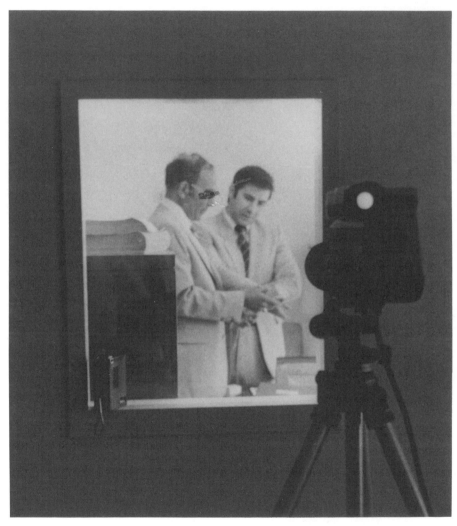

photo by David Holton
"Let me tell you a little bit about the way we work."

It seemed like a good question. Our attempt to answer it evolved into a case study of what was wrong with medicare and medicaid.

By 1982 the cost of the medicare program had increased from about $3 billion in 1967 to around $57 billion. There were three primary reasons for the increase: rampant and continuing fraud, waste, and abuse; inflation; and the increasing cost of care resulting from the development of new technologies.

The percentage of Americans receiving surgery increased from 37.5 percent in 1965 to 53.4 percent in 1981. This increase – known as the intensity factor – was the direct result of the development and use of technology and was said to account for as much as 25% of the increase in hospital costs.

Kidney transplants, hip replacements, artificial body parts, coronary bypass surgery, and new expensive diagnostic tools are examples of the technology that had evolved.

A decade before our investigation of clinical laboratories, we found automated labs had been developed that provided more than a dozen tests simultaneously for a fraction of the previous cost. The difference in some cases was as much as 300 percent. Yet, the government continued paying laboratories at the established rate.

It was enough of an incentive to encourage some entrepreneurs to start small labs, often in basements and garages, subcontract the tests to the automated facilities, and still net a handsome profit.

For at least twenty years, leading health care experts have called for systematic clinical trials to examine the cost, value, and effectiveness of new technologies, but no such system has evolved. As usual, the government's reaction was characterized by fragmenting responsibility to numerous organizations with limited scope and authority.

Until 1981, the Health Care Financing Administration had at least a limited capacity to examine technologies through the National Center for Health Care Technology. In the three years of its existence, it had determined that 40 percent of the technologies it evaluated were ineffective and without benefit to the patient.

Medicare refused to cover these technologies as a result of the center's evaluations. Harvard's School of Public Health estimated the center had saved the taxpayer somewhere between $100 million and $200 million through its evaluation of six technologies alone.

The center, never fully staffed, had been disbanded by the Reagan administration in its first run of cost cuts. The justifications were in part budget related and in part philosophical. The administration was convinced that the marketplace was a better laboratory for the evaluation of new technologies than any scientific center.

Among those questioning the wisdom of this decision was Arnold Relman, editor of the *New England Journal of Medicine*. Dr. Relman estimated at least 15 to 20 percent of the cost of health care could be saved if medical equipment was adequately tested and evaluated.

As an example, Relman cited a recent study by the National Institutes of Health, which had conducted a massive investigation of the proper indications for coronary bypass surgery years after the procedure was approved. NIH concluded at least 15 percent of those who had had the surgery probably didn't need it.

A similar study conducted at Harvard in 1982 was less conservative. The medical school review concluded two-thirds of the 110,000 bypass operations performed each year were unnecessary.

Radical mastectomy for breast cancer and routine tonsillectomy are two other recent examples of costly procedures now rarely performed as the result of clinical trials. The number of tonsillectomies has been reduced by over half a million in the last ten years. At cost of $1,000 each, the savings are significant.

We added up the cost of all tests, procedures, drugs, devices, employed in the treatment of disease that are not worth the money we spend on them, and we estimated that something in excess of $20 billion a year was being wasted as a result of ignorance or greed on useless and redundant procedures.

The pacemaker investigation presented us with a rare opportunity to document that fact and demonstrate the relation of the intensity and fraud factors. It also demonstrated the increasing institutionalization of corruption.

We were no longer talking about isolated instances of relatively small thefts by individuals on the fringes of the system. We were now faced with fraud that was bone-deep – endemic, institutionalized abuse that involves significant segments of the established medical community.

Six multi-national, billion dollar companies controlled 95 percent of the pacemaker industry. All of them were engaged in a consistent premeditated pattern of fraud and abuse. Fraud had become a standard business practice. It was mainline, expected, and accepted.

In the prophetic words of Joe Ingber, "Everybody was doing it."

We reviewed technical papers and professional journals concerning the development of pacemakers. Then we examined corporate reports of the six companies that controlled the pacemaker industry and examined the projections of market analysts.

With the help of the General Accounting Office, we audited bills submitted to medicare for 2,500 pacemakers that had been implanted over a two-year period. We also examined the records of four government agencies that share responsibility for regulating aspects of the pacemaker industry within medicare: the Federal Trade Commission, the Veterans Administration, the Securities and Exchange Commission, and the Food and Drug Administration.

We learned that medicare paid more than $2 billion annually for some 150,000 pacemaker operations a year, follow-up care, and monitoring of the half a million pacemaker patients. As much as half of the total, or $1 billion, was being wasted or stolen.

Many of the pacemaker procedures were unnecessary. Physicians we consulted indicated anywhere from 30 to 50 percent of the pacemaker implants were not needed.

A pacemaker that cost $600 to $900 to manufacture was sold to hospitals for $2,000 to $5,000. The hospitals, without any correlating expense, were increasing the cost by 50 to 150 percent and passing the total on to medicare.

Not surprisingly, this fat profit margin had encouraged the development of all kinds of creative marketing devices. Kickbacks, consulting fees, and other illegal arrangements were common.

Doctors were given everything from direct cash ($150 to $250 per pacemaker) to stock options in the company, payments for clinical evaluations (up to $25,000), vacations in the Caribbean, fishing excursions in Alaska and the Gulf of Mexico, gambling junkets, expensive gifts (gold plated shotguns, Rolex watches, and Australian opals, etc.), and all kinds of pacemaker accessories as an inducement to do business.

All of this, of course, was being added to the taxpayer's tab.

"The industry is totally unconcerned about price," one salesman said. "Couldn't care less. Medicare reimburses everything and they just don't care. God bless them, I love it."

"What about the doctors?"

"I thought doctors were something special until I started hanging around the doctor's lounge. They're no different from anybody else. It takes years before they can start earning and then they want to make as much as they can."

The problems we found in the pacemaker industry were notorious and of long standing. Five government agencies (the General Accounting Office, the Securities and Exchange Commission, the Veterans Administration, the Federal Trade Commission, and the Federal Bureau of Investigation) and committees of both houses of Congress had previously investigated and reported on some part of the pacemaker industry.

Yet, the problems persisted.

Faced with a staggering array of abuses, persistent allegations of criminality, and the potential for significant losses to the medicare program, we had arranged to go undercover.

Posing as the purchasing agents for a geriatric facility, we called representatives of the six major pacemaker firms to express our interest in getting involved in the business. The salesman in New York was one of sixteen we interviewed and one of six we filmed.

"We won't charge you for the paperwork or to train someone how to set up the clinic, because obviously no doctor is going to sit by the telephone all day."

"How long does it take?"

"Five minutes. Not even five minutes."

"How much can I bill for that?"

"You bill $200. It's unbelievable. You can make one-quarter of a million dollars a year doing this."

"For how many patients?"

"Around 400. I know a group here in Brooklyn that has 400 pacemaker patients, 400 that they are following. They take in well over one-quarter of a million dollars just with monitoring."

"Sounds easy."

"It's very easy. A nurse can do sixteen an hour very easily. And you're not paying anything. I mean stamps."

"Stamps."

"You have to pay stamps, right? Because you are sending it in the mail. That's basically it."

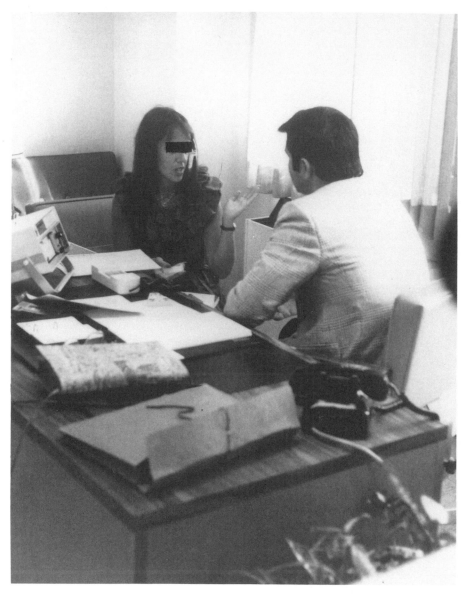

"All it will cost you is stamps!"   *photo by David Holton*

There was a microphone in the potted plant on the desk and a camera behind a one-way mirror on his right.

"Programmers we provide free of charge. If you need one, two, or three we provide those for you."

Programmers sell for $2,500 and are used to adjust the operating parameters of a pacemaker.

"Do you have a basic system analyzer?"

"No."

"It costs $3,500. If we do business we can get you one."

The salesman was on a roll, eager to be of service.

"I'll also go into the operating room with you. I'll do all the measurements. I'll scrub up and I'll go in with you. I can help coax you along in placing the leads."

"Anything else that we should know?"

"Are you a cardiologist?"

"No."

"Have you ever implanted a pacemaker?"

"No."

"We can send you out to California and train you to put in pacemakers yourself, but don't tell any surgeons I told you that. That's a political thing and I'm getting myself in trouble."

"How long does it take?"

"Fifteen minutes, if everything goes well."

"1 meant the training."

"Oh. Three or four days."

"How difficult is it?"

"The training?"

"The procedure."

"It's relatively easy. Fifteen minutes and they bill $2,100 – between $1,500 and $2,100."

The salesman seemed impressed. I sensed a little envy.

"Any pacemaker salesman will do anything for you. Face it, prices aren't that different. What it comes down to is service. We do anything you can think of and if you can think of it and we aren't doing it, we'll start."

"So there is absolutely nothing in terms of money out to you?"

The value of his "gifts" totalled $30,000.

"What we want is for your doctors to use our pacemakers as much as possible."

"What are we talking about in terms of cost?"

"The top of the line costs about $4,100."

"What's the bottom?"

"About $2,800."

I told him we were starting a health maintenance organization and had to be concerned about cost.

"Is that the best you can do?" I asked.

You could tell it was a question he didn't get often. He had to think about it.

"How many units are we talking about?"

"Over the course of a year, maybe twenty-five."

"I would say a discount of 15 percent would be the minimum you could expect."

Others had been more generous. We had been offered discounts of up to 50 percent. In most cases, the discounted price included all the "extras."

"And," concluded the salesman, "we pride ourselves on follow-up. With our no-hassle warranty, if you replace a competitor's product with ours, we give you a $450 credit."

Mrs. Garman had just turned eighty-nine when she appeared before our committee. Lawton Chiles, then the ranking Democrat on the Budget Committee, took pleasure in introducing his constituent.

"I still cannot understand why medicare should be paying for that pacemaker," Mrs. Garman said.

The day before we had played our New York tapes in an executive session. For years, we had acted as the committee's eyes and ears. With growing frustration, we had watched what was happening to our health system. We thought maybe it was time for them to see what we had seen.

The message had not been lost. Every member of the committee was present.

We had also released a carefully edited excerpt to ABC's "20/20." The Senate Caucus Room was packed.

Half way through the executive session Pete Domenici, Chairman of the Budget Committee, had slapped the table in disgust.

"You know that's just what's happening across the board. They're all doing it to us."

Pete had been with us since he was first elected to the Senate. He had participated in most of our hearings and joined us in the field for a first-hand look at clinical laboratories and medicaid mills. His frustration was evident.

"Cost-based reimbursement is at the core of this problem," he said.

The happy salesman's observation that "the industry is totally unconcerned about price" had stuck in his mind.

"That salesman was right. We have created a law that could care less about cost and, as a result, encourages everyone to get on the gravy train."

David Durenberger, Chairman of the Finance Committee's Health Subcommittee agreed.

"We can dump on the manufacturers, we can dump on the salesmen, we can sic the FBI on them, and we can have task forces coming out our ears at HHS, but the heart of the problem is right here, on this side of the green table."

Two weeks earlier a member of his staff, John Tillotson, had asked to see me. I had been expecting him. The largest pacemaker manufacturer is located in Minnesota. The company was known to be politically active and sophisticated. SEC records we'd pulled in phase one of the investigation had indicated an impressive range of contributions. Having learned our lesson, we were ready for them.

Without being asked, I took Tillotson through the investigation by the numbers. It took the better part of an hour. When I was done, almost as an afterthought, I mentioned we'd given the story to "20/20."

Tillotson is no dummy. He asked if I would brief Durenberger personally on

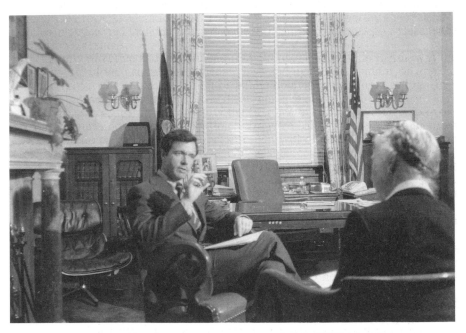

photo by Bill Halamandaris
Senator Heinz with consumer advisor Esther Peterson during the pacemaker investigation.

our findings.

"It's too bad it takes this kind of attention for us to look at the heart of the problem," Durenberger said at the hearing, "which is the way we reimburse for health care."

Senator Charles Grassley took a different tack.

Noting that many of the witnesses who were about to testify belonged to associations that lobby actively on a wide range of legislative issues, Grassley said, "Nothing could be less rewarding, less useful, than to hear only a parade of excuses, buck-passing and the tired explanation that, 'There are only a few isolated cases of abuse.'"

Grassley encouraged the lobbies to look inward.

"This committee has provided the examining room and now it is up to the physician to 'heal thyself.'"

John Heinz, the committee's chairman, picked up the most remarkable aspect of the investigation.

"We listened to hours of these tapes and it struck me as odd that all we heard was talk of how much money you could make and how little concern, if any, there was to what benefit there might be for the patient."

Most of the witnesses following Madeline Garman confirmed our findings, though some of the lobbyists could not bring themselves to be brave enough to follow Grassley's advice. But it was the industry's reaction that I found most interesting.

Despite the years of evidence and all the previous investigations, they seemed genuinely surprised. Russell Chambers, president of Intermedics, one of the largest manufacturers, noted our reference to the previous investigations by the SEC, the FTC, the VA, and the GAO.

"If, in fact, the problems are so acute, we have seen nothing from these agencies indicating severe problems."

At the break, Chambers and one of the hired guns who would subsequently go door to door peddling a rebuttal, asked for a few moments of my time. They were concerned about next steps.

I indicated the investigation was over. We had made our recommendations to the department and turned over all evidence to the FBI.

Chambers responded he was not concerned about the pacemaker industry. That damage had already been done. He was concerned about the rest of his product line.

He had cause.

In the seven previous years, his firm had increased revenues by a hundredfold. Profits had increased from $350,000 to $17 million.

By the time the other shoe had dropped, *Business Week* would pronounce the company "in critical condition" as a result "searing public scrutiny." Profits evaporated. Shares decreased in value from forty dollars to ten dollars.

Pacesetter, one of Intermedics competitors, fared even less well. The company plead guilty to charges of paying kickbacks of up to $175,000 to physicians who purchased the company's pacemakers. The company's former president and one of its regional sales managers also entered guilty pleas.

Chapter Nine
The Waterbed Principle
—— ❦ ——

The waterbed principle is a restatement of Newton's second law of motion. For every action, there is an equal and opposite reaction.

Following the pacemaker inquiry, Congress fashioned the most significant revision of the medicare program in its seventeen-year history. Congress established a prospective reimbursement system for hospitals.

Almost exactly a year before the reform, we had focused on the specific problem of hospital reimbursement for the thirtieth time in fifteen years. We had as one example a hospital in Perris, California.

Fourteen people had died in the hospital's six-bed intensive care unit in less than six weeks. All of them were elderly. All of them were poor. One of them was a 79-year-old woman who had walked into the hospital and was dead two hours later.

The Perris Valley Hospital presented a graphic example of what was wrong. The hospital was little more than a shell. Every service was contracted out to other related parties in a series of interrelated, self-serving deals designed to magnify the profit of a small band of businessmen.

Their sweetheart contracts created medicare charges for the hospital far in excess of average. In every case, the hospital's charges were greater than 90 percent of the hospitals participating in the program. In some cases Perris Valley's charges were 500 to 1,200 percent greater.

In total, we estimated that the combine had run $4.3 million through their subsidiaries, added 10 percent, and billed the total to the hospital. The hospital, doing nothing more, added 40 percent, and billed it to medicare. The hospital's add-on amounted to $3.5 million. Medicare, of course, paid it without question.

What we got for our money, according to the California Health Department, was substandard care. The Health Department charged the hospital had not hired enough people and engaged in "conduct inimical to the health and welfare of the hospital's patients." They were trimming the candle at both ends. People died as a result.

Senator Heinz summed up our findings, "The entrepreneurs who controlled this facility were too busy milking medicare to care about the people they were supposed to serve. It's way past time we re-examine the way we pay for services under medicare," Heinz concluded. "It's time we find a way to provide the incentives that will maximize service instead of maximizing reimbursement."

In light of the Perris Valley hearing and the years we'd spent criticizing medicare's pass-through reimbursement system you might have thought we would be clicking our heels with joy as a prospective payment system for hospitals approached. You would have been wrong.

It wasn't that we opposed the direction. Nor were we afraid the change would solve all our problems and leave us nothing to do. It was the waterbed principle. After a while you learn if you push down here, they'll pop up there.

Most of the continuing problems of the medicare and medicaid programs were predictable. Unfortunately, its architects had not bothered to examine the incentives they were creating. They didn't anticipate and prepare for the predictable reaction of the doctors, hospitals, nursing homes, and insurance companies. They were not prepared to monitor quality and prevent abuse.

Now, in attempting to solve the problem, we were repeating the process that created the problem.

The prospective plan divided hospital procedures into categories and reimbursed procedures on the average established for each category. Each bucket is called a diagnostic related group or DRG.

Hospitals that can deliver services for less than the established average are told they can keep the difference. Those who exceed the average are told they have to absorb the loss.

The administration estimated the plan would save $1.5 billion in 1984 and over $20 billion by 1989.

We had our doubts.

Prospective reimbursement isn't new. We all knew, or should have known, the kind of incentives it would create. In 1978 the owners of the Glendale Convalescent Center in Milwaukee were indicted for reckless conduct and neglect of fifty-eight mental patients. The charge was upped to homicide when one of the fifty-eight patients died.

The prosecutors said the owners had deliberately withheld food and limited the number of caregivers they hired in order to maximize their profits. The nursing home, like most of the nursing homes we investigated, was prospectively reimbursed. Whatever they didn't spend on patient care, they were allowed to keep.

Through the early 1970s we had chased a string of similar abuses related to health maintenance organizations. The concept was and is a good one – a flat fee to subscribers for all services.

With effort and the proper incentives any idea can be corrupted. In this case, the sharks and the wise guys moved in to maximize enrollment – in some cases, forging signatures and using strong-arm tactics. Once the patients were enrolled, they generally found it difficult to obtain service.

So now, though the party line was to do nothing to derail the progress of the prospective reimbursement process, we felt the need to remind people of what might happen.

It seemed appropriate to pull our example out of the nursing home environment, the place where extensive fraud, waste, and abuse were first evident. We focused on a Texas nursing home known as Autumn Hills.

A Galveston County grand jury had indicted the corporation that owned the nursing home and nine of its employees for murder. The attorney who had prepared the indictments, David Marks, told us the deaths were the result of poor care.

The poor care was said to be the result of greed. The owners of the corporation had established a corporate policy maximizing profits by limiting expenses. Two grand juries agreed. They found the nursing home had limited and withheld essential services, like nutritional supplements and medication.

Since the nursing home was paid on a prospective rate, the result was to extend the company's profit margin. Fifty-six patients were said to have died over a two-year period as a result.

The indictment charged they had reduced nursing personnel at the home and reduced the amount of food available to patients in order to maximize their profit. In this context, we asked the administration if it was prepared to deal with the incentives created by the new payment process for hospitals. To focus the discussion we released a copy of a confidential memo describing the New Jersey demonstration program on which the DRG system was modeled.

The memo came from Regional Administrator William Toby. Toby warned that the region's experience with "this complex and innovative reimbursement system has provided a number of valuable lessons for our policymakers." He warned of the need to guard against windfall profits at the expense of the taxpayer and the beneficiaries and to guard against the manipulation of secondary diagnoses and the provision of ancillary services in order to maximize reimbursement.

Within the demonstration period, according to Toby, hospitals had already designed computer programs to "determine the DRG for each patient, as originally reported, and then redetermine the DRG by reversing the first and second diagnoses."

The result was that audits of twenty hospitals in the first year of the demonstration had found that reimbursement had increased 16.3 percent while cost had only increased 9.7 percent.

An analysis of second-year demonstration costs of forty-one hospitals reimbursed under the new system found that they were reimbursed $30.9 million more than they would have been under the traditional medicare payment system.

Finally, the memo focused on the question of quality assurance. "If carried to the extreme," Toby said, "incentives exist in this system to manipulate ancillaries in order to maximize reimbursement. Similarly, premature discharges could occur to maximize reimbursement." He concluded, "A system that introduces such an incentive requires a focused quality assurance program."

Substantial as these concerns were, they were lost like whispers in the wind. In heated testimony, the administration told us they had read the memo and knew what they were doing. Only minor modifications were made to the prospective payment package.

In the following year, hospitals averaged a 15 percent profit margin, triple their average profit margin in the preceding years. For-profit hospitals did better than average, earning an 18 percent profit margin, and the phrase "sicker and quicker" was born.

Hospital administrators were pressured to release patients inside of the break-even point for each DRG established by medicare. One of those released early was Elsie McIntyre. Elsie was admitted for a stroke and uncontrolled diabetes in 1984. After a few days the 88-year-old woman was told she would have to leave because her medicare coverage had run out.

Frank Johnson, a 68-year-old Idaho man, was another. He was discharged after surgery with less than a day's notice, even though he lived more than 100 miles away and was still passing blood.

Patients with more than one chronic condition were soon being run through a revolving door of admission and release so that hospitals could collect payment for each diagnosis separately. One of these was an 86-year-old man with chronic heart and renal failure. He died after several hospital transfers.

Floyd Lane was admitted to a western hospital with a urinary tract infection, pneumonia, and chest pains. After two weeks, he was sent to a nursing home, then rushed back to the hospital two days later. He died in the emergency room.

Over 5,000 such abuses were reported in the first year of the new program. Twelve percent of the people who obtained hospital care said they were discharged too soon.

Almost as aggravating as the increasing evidence of patient manipulation by the hospitals is the knowledge that the government had institutionalized the fraud, waste, and abuse of the past. The payment rates for the new DRGs relied on the accuracy of the existing medicare data base.

A review of the respiratory charges of thirty-three hospitals, for example, found that the inappropriate data used to determine costs had overstated the hospitals' respiratory costs by 38 percent. By 1986, hospital charges were increasing at a ten times the rate of inflation. The consumer price index rose 1.9 percent in 1986. The cost of a hospital stay surged 19 percent.

The reason cited for the increase was that there were fewer patients, which forced hospitals to allocate the costs of a smaller base. In three-fifths of our states, the average hospital bed was empty as often as it was occupied.

There was also evidence that hospitals were trying to maximize the revenues generated by the smaller pool of patients by heaping on extra charges for tests and supplies. The biggest single increase in hospital charges was for ancillary services, like drugs, lab fees, and bandages.

During the pacemaker investigation a California salesman had added a sweetener.

"In addition, we sell intraocular lenses, heart valves, orthopedic devices, and other health products for seniors," he said. "We have great flexibility. We [the distributor] give. They [the manufacturer] give. We can even work out a package deal. We can arrange at least a 15 percent discount over VA approved prices." VA prices are 10 to 15 percent under medicare's prices.

Intraocular lenses are used in cataract surgery, the most common surgical procedure under medicare. Over a million lenses were implanted in 1985. The total cost of these procedures was over $3.5 billion. Medicare paid all but $500,000 of the total.

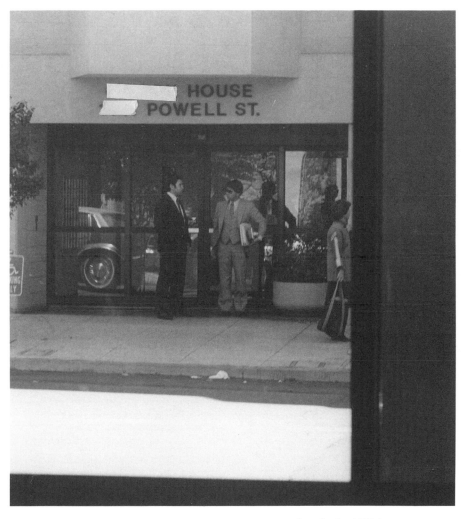

"We have great flexibility."

photo by David Holton

In 1981, before the advent of DRGs, cataract surgery was said to require a three-day hospital stay. In 1985, it took three hours and was done on an outpatient basis.

One would think that's what was intended when the prospective system was developed: reduced hospital stays would result in significant savings that could be passed on to medicare. Unfortunately, they hadn't allowed for the waterbed principle. The "significant savings" that resulted from the reduced hospital stays became increased profits medicare never saw.

Under the DRG payment system, medicare paid $2400 for cataract surgery when performed in the hospital. The same procedure, performed by the same hospital on an outpatient basis – using only three hours of the hospital's resources – costs medicare more, not less. We found the average outpatient cost billed to medicare for this procedure was more than twice the inpatient cost and as much as $5,700.

The cost of manufacturing the lense implants was said to be thirty-five to fifty dollars. In 1981, the average cost to medicare was $285. In 1985 lenses purchased for inpatient use under competitive bidding were available for $100 or less. Lenses purchased for outpatient use were bought under the old rules and billed to the medicare program at a "reasonable cost" of $325 to $500 a piece.

Under the old rules, the old inducements still prevailed. Doctors were being bought with inducements ranging from cash ($50 a lense implant), to stock in the company, "free" lasers, and other equipment.

One manufacturer instituted a "buy-one-get-one-free" policy. Of course, you billed medicare for both.

In Texas, where they do everything with style, a surgeon received 1,600 "free" lenses. He charged medicare $54,000 for them. It was only part of the $1.3 million he had received from the government for implanting lens in 1984.

"Medicare is saying to you, 'Here is your $500, or your $490, or whatever reimbursement,'" one salesman said. "'Go out and do whatever you can, get your best deal.'"

A second salesman added, "The other thing is you're aware of the way it is around here – they don't look at invoices. They have a set charge they allow. They don't say, 'Well, we won't pay as much because you only paid $300 for that lens.' They don't look at that."

By the time we had backed out the exorbitant profits, the kickbacks, and the hospital cost-shifting games, we were where we had started. As much as half of medicare's cataract expenditures were unnecessary.

"The whole system is corrupt and it's corrupting physicians," one ophthalmologist said.

He was right.

We now spend more than 12 percent of our gross national product on health – twice what we spent when medicare and medicaid were enacted. We spend more and get less than any developed nation in the world.

Sweden, France, Canada, West Germany, and the United Kingdom all spend less than 10 percent of their GNP on health – some of them far less. All of these countries provide comprehensive health care for all of their citizens. We provide limited services for parts of our society.

One quarter of our increase is related to technology and the intensity of services. Americans are four times as likely to have a coronary bypass operation than western Europeans and twice as likely as Canadians with the same symptoms.

The reason isn't medical. It's financial. A surgeon who performs two to three bypass operations a week will earn more than $300,000 a year.

As recently as 1937, as Dr. Lewis Thomas has pointed out, the essence of medical practice was custodial. There was little that could be done to alter the course of infectious disease beyond good nursing care. The practice of medicine was "accepted to be a chancy way to make a living, and nobody expected a doctor to get rich, least of all the doctors themselves."

Now most people entering the medical profession expect to be rich or at least live very well. The practice of nursing, "caring" for people has been delegated to nurses, aides, and therapists.

Average income for all physicians was around $150,000 in 1987. It was $28,960 in 1965 and had doubled in the first ten years of medicare and medicaid to $58,440.

In 1965 there were about 277,000 doctors in America. Today, there are nearly twice that number. We have gone from one doctor for every 700 Americans to one for every 470. It's estimated that within two years we will have a surplus of at least 70,000 physicians and as many as 185,000.

The big fear in the early 1960s was something called "socialized medicine," whatever that is. We have fallen prey to something worse – industrialized medicine. The entire focus of our health care system has shifted from social, ethical, and moral considerations to those of finance, economy, and business.

Physicians no longer "care for people." Caring for people is old-fashioned and unprofitable. Caring involves thinking, talking, touching, counseling, and becoming involved with patients. These "social" and "cognitive services" are unprofitable. What pays off are procedures.

Anything that involves cutting, jabbing, or injecting is called a "procedure" and is far more profitable. Surgeons average $1,000 an hour. If the same surgeon spends an hour counseling a patient, he will be lucky if he can bill for $50. In other words, we have made what a doctor does to you more profitable than what he can do for you.

Not surprisingly, the number of procedures billed under medicare and medicaid has increased geometrically. Within two years of the enactment of the federal programs, an investigation by the Senate Finance Committee found that "many physicians are now billing separately for services like laboratory tests, which were previously routinely included in a charge for an office visit or surgical fee."

This fact helps explain one of the most startling statistics in this book: the number of physician visits for the elderly has actually not increased since the introduction of medicare. The average number of physician visits per person in 1970 was 6.3. In 1980 it was 6.4. However, the number of physician bills submitted to medicare has exploded from 1,690 to 4,260 per 1,000 beneficiaries in the same time period.

Many of these procedures are clearly unnecessary. A sister committee of the

House estimated in 1974 that 2.4 million unnecessary surgeries were performed at a cost of $4 billion and nearly 12,000 lives.

No parallel study has been done in recent years. But the Inspector General's Office, which has been lobbying for a policy mandating second opinions for elective surgery, estimates that such a policy would reduce the number of operations in medicaid by 29 percent. The same policy would reduce medicare surgeries by 18 percent. The combined dollar savings for the two programs would be at least $150 million.

Our infatuation with the glittering gadgets of modern medicine have fueled the increase in the intensity of services. It may also have contributed to a reduction in the quality of medicine.

Most of the technology developed over the last twenty years has been designed to help diagnose illness. CAT scans and ultrasound imaging are only the most visible and expensive examples.

Despite this marvelous machinery, the accuracy of physicians' diagnoses may have actually declined over the last twenty years. A 1983 Harvard study assessed the accuracy of diagnoses over the last twenty years by comparing diagnoses with autopsy reports. The researchers concluded that while diagnostic tools have been getting better, diagnoses have been getting worse. Doctors had missed problems that might have been treated and prolonged life in 8 percent of the cases reviewed in 1960. That number had increased to 10 percent in 1980.

A clue as to what may be happening is provided by studies of pap tests. Pap tests are used to detect cervical cancer or precursor cell abnormalities. Each year 60,000 women develop cervical cancer and about 7,000 die from it.

Pap tests have been effective and have helped reduce deaths from cervical cancer. But over the years, they have earned the reputation as being among the most inaccurate of all clinical laboratory procedures. Studies have shown pap test results have been inaccurate in at least 20 percent and as many as 40 percent of all cases.

The pap test involves smearing cells from the cervix on a slide. A study by the American College of Obstetricians and Gynecologists indicated physicians had not performed this simple process adequately in at least 50 percent of the cases. In other words, the lab errors that resulted were not the fault of the laboratory process, but rather the result of inadequate cell specimens obtained by physicians.

The failure of physicians to master this relatively simple process confounded the study group. Caught in the irony of a refined and improved technology producing diminishing results, the college concluded that "after thirty years of physician education, this effort has been spectacularly unsuccessful."

The head of a local lab confirmed the college's conclusion and provided a clue: "Some of the best pap smears we get come from non-physicians, like nurse practitioners," he said. "They simply take the time and want to do a good job."

These things make it easier to understand how a graduate of a cartoon college in the Caribbean or some other checkbook doctor can practice for years without discovery. Sometimes it's hard to tell the good guys from the bad guys.

It also puts the raging controversy over medical malpractice in context. Ten years ago, three out of every 100 physicians were sued. Now the number is up to one out of every five. The average award was $166,165 in 1974. It had increased tenfold to $1,179,095 by 1985.

Understandably, the medical lobby has been screaming for years that physicians need some protection from malpractice claims. Guaranteed the good life, status, income, and freedom from criminal prosecution, the civil courts are their last point of vulnerability – and then only if they should injure or antagonize a middle-class patient.

When you're dealing with medicare and medicaid the only one who gets sued is the government. Doctors have no reason to be afraid. The elderly are said to make poor witnesses and often don't live long enough to survive the court process. If they should sue and win, the measure of damages will be limited by their age.

The poor simply don't sue.

It's a bit inconsistent for doctors to lobby for protection from their patients. What is inconsistent is the argument, not the objective.

Organized elements of the medical community, most visibly the American Medical Association, have managed to be against nearly every progressive health measure that has come before the public in the last quarter of a century. Medicare, utilization reviews, vaccines, and public inoculations have all been opposed on the hallowed grounds that the adoption of these public health measures would interfere with the sanctity of the relationship between physicians and their patients.

The AMA's opposition to medicare was substantial enough that President Kennedy was forced to qualify his request to Congress for the program with the promise:

"This program is not a program of socialized medicine. It is a program of prepayment of health costs with absolute freedom of choice guaranteed. No service performed by any physician at either home or in the office, no fee he charges for such services would be involved, covered, or affected in any way. There would be no supervision or control over the practice of medicine by the doctor or over the manner in which medical services are provided by any hospital."

Small wonder the costs of the program have skyrocketed. Few things are more attractive than the thought of spending someone else's money.

The AMA also opposed the creation of Inspector General's Office, designed to lock up crooked doctors. You would think they would have the same reason every other citizen has to be concerned about these abuses and then some, but through the years they have been consistent. Their reaction to our investigations of racketeering, embezzlement, theft, fraud, and homicide has been to minimize, deny, and remember come election day.

I've always thought we should have received some sort of a campaign contribution finder's fee. Whoever we worked for could always count on a few dollars from the medical community to "keep the door open."

Unfortunately, his opponent could count on several times that. The AMA's revenge for the creation of the Inspector General's Office, for example, was to get an assist in the defeat of Senator Moss, our first chairman. Moss' opponent benefited extensively from the generosity of the medical community.

Despite the inescapable evidence the program is coming apart at its seams, the AMA remained consistent in its dogged pursuit of economic advantage and self-interest. In July of 1977, they were asked by the Senate Finance Committee to come up with some cost-reduction options that might be more palatable than those then under consideration by Congress. The AMA came up with a list of twelve suggestions. All of them would have increased the cost of care to the beneficiaries. As someone once said, a lot of things go round in the dark besides Santa Claus.

Now the AMA is lobbying for legislation that would limit physician liability. They have asked the states and federal government to cap the amount the courts can award, and some states have agreed.

What they haven't done is to try and clean up their own mess. In Pennsylvania, 25 percent of malpractice payments are the result of the actions of 1 percent of the practicing physicians. Nationwide, the experience is similar.

Yet only 406 medical licenses were revoked in 1985 in the United States. All of the 1700 others received formal rebukes. Checkbook doctors and known incompetents have been allowed to practice and continue practicing despite criminal activity, unethical conduct, and patient abuse.

The medical community achieved its standing based on a perception of service to society. It began with the Hippocratic oath and the selflessness that implied. In this generation, medical practice has shifted from being among the most selfless to being among the most selfish of professions. Lured by the changing perception of the nature of medical practice, too many hypocrites are taking the Hippocratic oath.

Evidence can be found in surveys of the social commitment of those entering various professions. Once physicians would have ranked first in terms of social commitment. They now come in well down the list, somewhere below engineers and above lawyers.

It is sad, but not surprising therefore, to read that 25 percent of recent medical school graduates do not feel obligated to care for AIDS victims.

Primary responsibility resides with the medical societies established to defend the status of their profession. By and large, they have not served their masters well, interpreting protection as defense and defining status in economic terms.

In August of 1986, Edward J. Kuriansky, the Deputy Attorney General for Medicaid Fraud Control in New York, completed an undercover review of welfare clinics in New York. It was a reprise of the investigation we had conducted ten years earlier.

Kuriansky's people concluded entrepreneurs have taken over the industry. Public funds are "hemorrhaging" into the streets.

Thirty-four doctors and pharmacists were arrested. The people accused of ripping off the government had billed medicaid for $25 million in the previous two years.

In 1990 Kuriansky released a statement announcing the single largest medicaid fraud case ever prosecuted. The owners of a Brooklyn clinic, a father and two sons, had "systematically looted" the program to the tune of $13.3 million.

The owners were said to have been engaged in assembly-line medicine. They billed medicaid for hundreds of thousands of phantom patient visits. Prosecutors said they used the profit from their service to the poor to purchase a lifestyle that included two apartments in the Trump Tower on Fifth Avenue, a luxurious home in Boca Raton, Florida, expensive automobiles including a Rolls Royce, and other creature comforts.

It's not that the reforms of the last twenty years have had no impact. It's the waterbed principle. Many of the changes made have been helpful, but they have been too little, too late. They have been too specific in their focus and too immediate in their objective.

The problems that plague our health care system are endemic. They are broad and bone-deep. Any attempt to address part of the problem without addressing the context in which these problems develop is doomed to failure.

Chapter Ten
Prescription
——❦——

We are punished not so much for our sins as by them. In 1965 our primary concern was to guarantee access to health care for those most in need – the poor and the elderly. This access was purchased with the premise that doctors, hospitals, and other institutionalized providers would be given carte blanche.

The generosity of medicare and medicaid's reimbursement systems and the inescapable demands of human greed have fundamentally altered the nature of medicine in this country and the mentality of the men and women who practice medicine. The line between good medicine and good business has blurred, diminished, and occasionally disappeared.

Senator Moss once said, "Medicare and medicaid aren't medicine. They are business." This has increasingly become the case over the last twenty years.

Worse, as medicine has become business we have been left with a crisis in health care of major proportions. Our health system is at once bloated and incomplete. Billions are wasted yearly, yet millions are unserved.

Medicare has been approaching bankruptcy and continues to be in jeopardy despite the elimination of many benefits and the shifting of responsibility for billions of dollars in services to the backs of beneficiaries. Meanwhile, fraud, waste, and abuse continue unabated.

We have not socialized medicine so much as industrialized it. We have combined the worst aspects of a government program with the predatory instincts of the free market. As a result, it seems now hard to imagine that there was ever a time when ripping off our health programs was a novelty.

We have addressed individual problems incrementally, patching a patchwork program. What we haven't done is address the fundamental problem. There are too many cracks, too many holes, too little consistency, care, and control.

We do not have a health system. We have many health systems, each limited in purpose and audience. They are at once too little and too much, overlapping in some areas while leaving others entirely uncovered.

At the same time, we are confronted with the greatest threat to public health in 100 years. We have an epidemic of chronic illness approaching that will sorely test our health system, our ingenuity, and our national will.

The crisis is at once a challenge and an opportunity. It is likely to be the paramount political and moral test of our times. In order to meet this challenge we will have to radically reform the way we take care of sick people in this country. Our institutional bias will have to give way to community care, technology will have to leave room for humanity, acute care will have to expand to include chronic care, and fragmentation will have to be replaced by coordination.

Time and time again, people have said we can't move forward with a national health program until we clean this mess up. The fact is we will never clean up the mess until we move forward. There are too many cracks, too many layers of bureaucracy, too many places to hide.

For example, twenty-six programs pay for the care of chronically ill children in Arizona. Together they pay for something less than 70 percent of the cost of caring for these children.

What should we do?

Return to where we began. Recognize access to quality health care is a fundamental right and the moral obligation of society. It is the cornerstone on which all other social policies depend.

Eliminate the fragmentation of our current multi-faceted, multi-tiered health system. Begin with the premise that we will provide a basic level of quality health care to all of our people – the "what." Then quarrel about who will be responsible for what.

There is plenty of room for private enterprise, health insurers, and creative development. But these should be extensions of a basic policy, and that policy requires a national commitment that every man, woman, and child in this country will be assured access to quality health care when they are in need.

Need should be the fundamental criteria – not age, not income, not political persuasion, nor perceptions of some particular moral obligation to some segment of our society.

At minimum, the federal role should include the provision of services for those in greatest need – the poor and the elderly, the disabled – those Hubert Humphrey once said lived in the shadows of our society.

At minimum, the federal government's responsibility should include the creation and enforcement of national standards of quality and service, and the protection of the consumer and the taxpayer.

At minimum, the private sector is responsible for the health care of its work force.

How?

You have to play the hand you're dealt. Right now we have a system that is marked by inefficiency and excess: too many doctors (many of them marginal), too many hospitals, too many procedures, too much money being spent on the acute side, and negligence – the absence of significant services and appropriate resources for chronic care.

The surplus of providers gives us an opportunity to evaluate, select, and redirect providers and facilities. It also provides us with the opportunity to weed out the marginal players, increase efficiency, and redirect services.

What we have is a system that forces a patient into serious illness before it will pay, encouraging dependence, intensity of services, and institutionalization.

What we need is a paradigm shift, a new national health policy designed to maximize independence, minimize hospitalization, reduce the number of unnecessary or useless services required, and limit institutionalization.

Those who quarrel with the development of a national health program have done so historically on two grounds. They have argued that we either lack the capacity to organize an efficient and effective national health program, or that the creation of such a program will somehow corrupt our national values, leading us down to the road to socialism.

I refuse to believe that the United States is incapable of doing what nearly every other developed nation has done. I am chauvinist enough to believe we can do it better. As for the dangers of "socialized medicine" that is and always has been a straw man thrown up by the medical establishment to camouflage self-interest.

There is room for self-interest, but not at the expense of the public's interest. Unfortunately, that has been the public face of medicine over the past two dozen years. For those ideological purists who want to be concerned about the intrusion of government into our lives, I suggest the health system is not a point of particular vulnerability. The federal government's involvement in health is much less, for example, than in education. At its worst, a national health program would be nowhere near as intrusive and, should the evil empire appear, it is infinitely less corruptible and corruptive.

From my perspective, a fundamental revision of the way we care for people in this country is inevitable. We simply have no choice. My hope is that we have learned enough from the past to anticipate the natural consequences of our actions and their impact on the fabric of our society. Finally, we must come to accept the fact that every success carries the seeds of failure. Remembering the lessons of Douglas and the lawmakers of the Thurians, we must always be prepared to begin again.